Dermatology
pearls and pitfalls

Clinical Challenges for the Practitioner

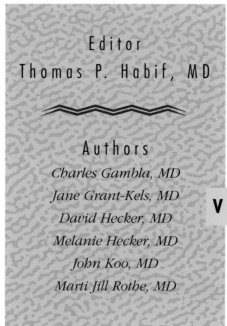

Editor
Thomas P. Habif, MD

Authors

Charles Gambla, MD

Jane Grant-Kels, MD

David Hecker, MD

Melanie Hecker, MD

John Koo, MD

Marti Jill Rothe, MD

Volume 2

Provided as an educational service by

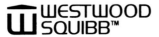WESTWOOD SQUIBB™

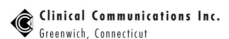Clinical Communications Inc.
Greenwich, Connecticut

Group Publisher: Corey Kupersmith, RPh
Publisher: Bradley D. Mock
Editorial Director: Lois Gandt
Project Editor: Diann Peterson
Art Director: Jill Ruscoll

Clinical Communications Inc.
Greenwich Office Park #6
Greenwich, CT 06830

ISBN: 1-57013-052-3

Printed in the United States of America

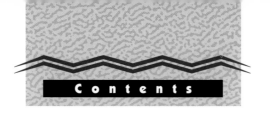

Contents

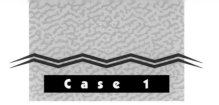

𝒞hief Complaint

Nonhealing ulcers on leg

ℋistory of the Present Illness

A 20-year-old woman with a lifelong history of recessive dystrophic epidermolysis bullosa complained of ulcers on the right leg that have not healed for the past 9 months. She has had no treatment except local wound care with bacitracin under Telfa® to erosions and ulcerations.

𝒫hysical Examination and Laboratory

Examination revealed a cachectic female with contraction deformities of both hands, blisters and ulcerations predominantly affecting the distal extremities, and hyperkeratotic nodules and exuberant granulation tissue within ulcerations of the right ankle.

Biopsies of the hyperkeratotic nodules and exuberant granulation tissue showed irregular masses of atypical keratinocytes extending into the dermis.

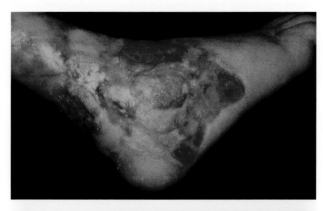

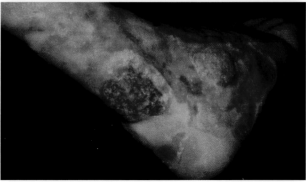

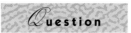

Question

*W*hat complications are associated with recessive dystrophic epidermolysis bullosa?

Discussion

Complications of recessive dystrophic epidermolysis bullosa include:

- Syndactyly and mitten deformities of the hands and feet;
- Contractures of the elbows, knees, ankles, and wrists;
- Secondary bacterial infection;
- Anemia;
- Gastrointestinal involvement;
- Nutritional compromise; and
- Squamous cell carcinoma arising in chronic ulcerations.

Nutritional compromise is multifactorial. Gingival disease and dental caries are common and can lead to tooth loss. Fragility of the oral mucosa and subsequent lingual adhesions and microstomia further impede food intake. Esophageal webs account for most complaints of dysphagia and occur as early as the first decade of life. Esophageal bullae and spasms also contribute to dysphagia. Deformities of the hands limit the ease of self-feeding. Extensive erosions and ulcerations can lead to protein malnutrition, which in turn, compromises wound healing. Intervention should include careful attention to dental hygiene, cautious dilatation of esophageal strictures, and nutritional supplementation. Gastrostomy feeding tubes have been advocated to ensure adequate intake.

Cutaneous squamous cell carcinomas, which can be difficult to detect clinically, not uncommonly arise in areas of chronic nonhealing ulceration or hyperkeratotic crusting. Pseudoepitheliomatous hyperplasia is a histopathologic feature that can occur at the edges of chronic ulcers and may be difficult to distinguish from squamous cell carcinomas. In patients with epidermolysis bullosa, squamous cell carcinomas typically develop on the extremities, have a high rate of metastases, and may lead to death. Early lesions can be treated with traditional surgical excision or Mohs' micrographic surgery; advanced lesions may necessitate amputation. Wound healing of excision sites may be difficult.

*C*linical Pearls and Pitfalls

1. Poor nutrition in patients with recessive dystrophic epidermolysis bullosa potentially can be ameliorated by special attention to dentition, esophageal stricture, and dietary supplementation. Dermatologists can play an important role in facilitating referral to dentists, gastroenterologists, and nutritionists with expertise to address the special needs of these patients.

2. Squamous cell carcinomas in patients with dystrophic epidermolysis bullosa can be difficult to detect, have a high rate of metastases, and may lead to death. Frequent surveillance and biopsy of chronic ulcerations and long-standing hyperkeratotic crusting are critical.

Suggested Readings

1. Birge K. Nutrition management of patients with epidermolysis bullosa. *J Am Dietetic Assoc*. 1995;95:575-579.
2. Dunnill MGS, Eady RAJ. The management of dystrophic epidermolysis bullosa. *Clin Exp Dermatol*. 1995;20:179-188.
3. Ergun GA, Lin AN, Dannenberg AJ, et al. Gastrointestinal manifestations of epidermolysis bullosa. A study of 101 patients. *Medicine*. 1992;71:121-127.
4. McGrath JA, Schofield OM, Mayou BJ, et al. Epidermolysis bullosa complicated by squamous cell carcinoma: Report of 10 cases. *J Cutaneous Pathology*. 1992;19:116-123.
5. Newman C, Wagner RF, Tyring SK, et al. Squamous cell carcinoma secondary to recessive dystrophic epidermolysis bullosa. A report of 4 patients with 17 primary cutaneous malignancies. *J Dermatol Surg Oncol*. 1992:18:301-305.
6. Travis SP, McGrath JA, Turnbull AJ, et al. Oral and gastrointestinal manifestations of epidermolysis bullosa. *Lancet*. 1992;340:1505-1506.
7. Wright JT, Fine JD, Johnson L. Hereditary epidermolysis bullosa: Oral manifestations and dental management. *Pediatric Dentistry*. 1993;15:242-248.

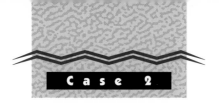

Chief Complaint

Generalized atopic dermatitis unresponsive to topical or systemic corticosteroids

History of the Present Illness

A 42-year-old Filipino-American woman with a 20-year history of atopic dermatitis presented at the Psoriasis Treatment Center. In the past, she had received various topical corticosteroid agents (up to the super-potency strength), intramuscular triamcinolone acetonide, oral prednisone, and various oral antibiotics and antihistamines, without obtaining any lasting benefits. She underwent extensive patch testing for possible contact allergies; these tests proved noncontributory. Family history was significant for a sister with atopic dermatitis who also had twin daughters with severe atopic dermatitis. The patient denied any childhood history of asthma, atopic dermatitis, or allergic rhinitis. She had been admitted as an inpatient for treatment of both exacerbation of atopic dermatitis and secondary cellulitis resulting from excoriation. By the time she was referred to the Center for possible phototherapy, including the Goeckerman regimen, she was almost suicidal because she was very frustrated with various therapies that seemed to give only temporary relief.

Physical Examination

The dry, eczematoid, pruritic lesions covered at least 80% of the patient's total body surface area. Her face was about the only site that had been spared. The patient had eczematoid involvement of her scalp; moreover, she had lichenifications on her back with numerous excoriations, which did not appear infected. Deep, violaceous striae on the back and shoulders secondary to chronic use of various topical steroids, including superpotent agents, also were noted.

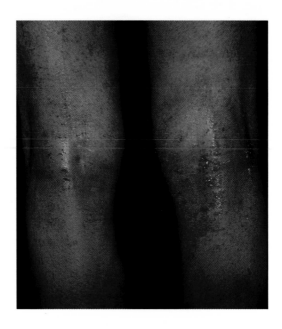

What are other treatment alternatives for patients with atopic dermatitis unresponsive to systemic or topical steroids and other usual outpatient treatment modalities?

*D*iscussion

Patients with atopic dermatitis respond at least as well to phototherapy and black tar as patients with psoriasis do. One of the reasons patients with atopic dermatitis do not receive phototherapy as frequently as steroids is because eczema tends to respond better than psoriasis to topical steroids. Also, systemic steroids, which are not generally recommended for treatment of psoriasis, can be given safely to patients with atopic dermatitis. However, if the dermatitis proves to be unresponsive to steroid therapy, it is important to consider the use of phototherapy, including outpatient UVB, systemic PUVA therapy, and the

Goeckerman regimen. Among these three options, the most effective mode of therapy may be traditional Goeckerman therapy.

This patient was admitted to the Psoriasis Day Treatment Program. Her entire body was covered with a thick application of 2% crude coal tar in petrolatum. Prior to the application of crude coal tar, she received UVB, starting at 10 millijoules, which was eventually raised to 40 millijoules by the end of the treatment session. In just 8 days of Goeckerman therapy, the atopic dermatitis cleared completely. The patient was able to maintain this improvement with outpatient UVB therapy three times per week and use of 20% liquor carbonis detergens (LCD) in Aquaphor® for the body and 20% LCD in Nutraderm® for the scalp; both are applied at bedtime and washed off in the morning.

Goeckerman therapy for atopic dermatitis differs from that for psoriasis in some important aspects. The concentration of tar is kept at 2% since higher concentrations such as 5% or 10% crude coal tar tend to be less lubricating because of decreased content of petroleum. Salicylic acid or lactic acid is not used since removing hyperkeratotic layers of the skin is not an issue. Lastly, phototherapy is conducted very carefully. Atopic dermatitis is treated as if the skin is type I; the intensity of the UVB application is increased gradually. Such application was necessary in this case, even though the patient's skin was type IV. Patients with atopic dermatitis are unusually sensitive to UVB, and it is not uncommon for the patient to experience phototherapy-induced burning or other irritation before a stable regimen is established. Phototherapy for patients with atopic dermatitis requires much more patience than that for patients with psoriasis. With attention to details and patience, it is generally possible to identify a regimen that works well, not only for short-term benefits but also for long-term control of the skin condition.

Even though LCD in Aquaphor ointment is widely used to treat psoriasis, patients with atopic dermatitis may be irritated by the Aquaphor ointment. This may very well be due to the wool alcohol content of the Aquaphor ointment. Sometimes, these patients tolerate petroleum. Other times, if the patient complains of sensitivity even to petroleum, tar may have to be formulated creatively. For example, black tar is sometimes compounded into a non-ionic base cream, which is an ammonium base that is commercially available and appears to be well tolerated by patients with atopic dermatitis undergoing Goeckerman therapy, either in a formal day treatment setting or as an outpatient.

$\mathscr{C}$linical Pearls and Pitfalls

1. Phototherapy works at least as well for atopic dermatitis and other forms of eczema as for psoriasis. It may turn out to be the treatment of choice for atopic dermatitis that does not respond to steroid therapy.

2. Among the various modes of phototherapy available, traditional Goeckerman therapy, modified for atopic dermatitis patients, tends to work better than PUVA therapy or simple outpatient UVB therapy.

3. Atopic dermatitis patients tend to be irritated by wool and ointment containing wool alcohol. Tar and LCD may have to be formulated in something other than Aquaphor ointment, such as petroleum or non-ionic base cream.

Suggested Readings

1. Cooper KD. New therapeutic approaches in atopic dermatitis. *Clin Rev Allergy.* 1993;11(4):543-559.

2. Jekler J. Phototherapy of atopic dermatitis with ultraviolet radiation. *Acta Dermato-Venereologica.* 1992;171(Suppl):1-37.

3. Jekler J, Larko O. Phototherapy for atopic dermatitis with ultraviolet A (UVA), low-dose UVB and combined UVA and UVB: two paired-comparison studies. *Photodermatology, Photoimmunology and Photomedicine.* 1991;4:151-156.

4. Morison WL. Phototherapy and photochemotherapy. *Adv Dermatol.* 1992;7:255-270.

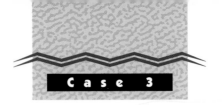

Case 3

*C*hief Complaint

Widespread redness and scaling

*H*istory of the Present Illness

A 55-year-old man with a long history of psoriasis affecting the elbows, knees, and scalp suddenly had a widespread flare of his disease. He failed to respond first to topical steroids and later to etretinate. He was otherwise in good health and was not receiving other medications.

*P*hysical Examination and Laboratory

Examination revealed widespread salmon-colored erythema and scaling, with rare areas of uninvolved skin, affecting the trunk, extremities, face, and neck. The periphery of plaques was remarkable for collarettes. No blisters, pustules, or erosions were evident. Ectropion was present. The scalp showed diffuse scaling; fingernails showed pitting. The patient was shivering.

Biopsy for routine histology of a red plaque with collarette of the arm showed a subcorneal pustule with acantholysis. Biopsy for direct immunofluorescence from uninvolved skin of the arm showed IgG and C3 deposited in the intercellular spaces. Biopsy for routine histology of a red plaque of the left hand showed acanthosis with parakeratosis, elongated papillae with tortuous blood vessels, and a superficial perivascular infiltrate in the papillae with polymorphonuclear leukocytes extending from the papillae to the epidermis.

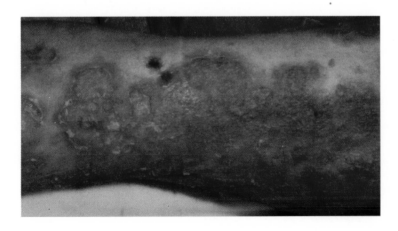

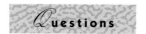

$\mathcal{W}$hat is the diagnosis?

$\mathcal{W}$hat is the differential diagnosis of erythroderma?

$\mathcal{W}$hat are the treatment options?

$\mathcal{D}$iscussion

A diagnosis of new-onset pemphigus foliaceus in a patient with a history of localized plaque psoriasis was made. Both conditions may manifest themselves as erythroderma. The differential diagnosis of erythroderma also includes atopic dermatitis, contact dermatitis, chronic actinic dermatitis, drug reactions, pityriasis rubra pilaris, cutaneous T-cell lymphoma, other lymphomas/leukemias and underlying internal malignancies, urticarial pemphigoid, and dermatomyositis; 10% to 25% of cases of erythroderma are considered idiopathic.

Determining the underlying cause of erythroderma relies on clinicopathologic correlation, as well as observations regarding response to therapy. Multiple biopsies from different anatomic areas and at different times during the course of the disease are helpful in augmenting the accuracy of histopathologic evaluation. Clinical features such as alopecia, keratoderma, and onychodystrophy are nonspecific manifestations related to chronicity of erythroderma. Erythroderma of acute onset of 3 days or less is relatively specific for drug reactions; resolution within 2 to 6 weeks also is suggestive of drug reactions. Often erythroderma can be attributed to a preexisting dermatosis; however, as in this case, the cause of erythroderma in a patient with preexisting skin disease should be reconsidered when treatment yields no improvement.

Baths, bland emollients, low-to-medium strength topical corticosteroids, and antihistamines are useful for the treatment of acute erythroderma. Ideally, chronic therapy is directed toward the underlying dermatosis. In this case, high-dose systemic corticosteroids were essential to gain rapid control of the pemphigus foliaceus; methotrexate was an effective steroid-sparing agent, which permitted gradual withdrawal of systemic steroids without flare of either the pemphigus or psoriasis. Cyclosporine also might have been effective therapy for coexisting pemphigus foliaceus and psoriasis.

*C*linical Pearls and Pitfalls

1. The diagnosis of the underlying cause of erythroderma requires clinicopathologic correlation and observation of response to treatment.

2. Multiple biopsies from different anatomic sites and at different points during the course of the disease are helpful in establishing a definitive diagnosis.

3. A history of a preexisting dermatosis is usually a critical clue in establishing the cause of erythroderma. However, failure to respond to therapy should prompt a search for a coexisting dermatosis or underlying malignancy.

Suggested Readings

1. Botella-Estrada R, Sammartin O, Oliver V, et al. Erythroderma. A clinicopathological study of 56 cases. *Arch Dermatol.* 1994;130:1503-1507.
2. King LE Jr. Erythroderma. Who, where, when, why, and how. *Arch Dermatol.* 1994;130:1545-1547.
3. Walsh NMG, Prokopetz R, Tron VA, et al. Histopathology in erythroderma: Review of a series of cases by multiple observers. *J Cutan Pathol.* 1994;21:419-423.
4. Wilson DC, Jester JD, King LE Jr. Erythroderma and exfoliative dermatitis. *Clin Dermatol.* 1993;11:67-72.
5. Zip C, Murray S, Walsh NMG. The specificity of histopathology in erythroderma. *J Cutan Pathol.* 1993;20:393-398.

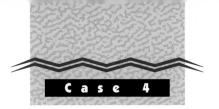

Chief Complaint

Generalized plaque psoriasis during pregnancy

History of the Present Illness

A 40-year-old woman, whose pregnancy was at 21 weeks' gestation, presented at the Psoriasis Center complaining of generalized psoriasis. She reported a 17-year history of plaque-like psoriasis. Her father also had a history of severe psoriasis. The patient's medical history was significant for four spontaneous miscarriages, possibly due to a bicornuate uterus. She underwent corrective surgery for the bicornuate uterus with an apparently successful outcome. Prior to discovering that she was pregnant, the patient had been treating her psoriasis with 20% liquor carbonis detergens (LCD) in Aquaphor® and mometasone furoate cream. When she found out that she was pregnant, she stopped using the mometasone furoate cream. The patient had no other active medical problems.

Physical Examination and Laboratory

General physical examination showed a positive gravid uterus at approximately 22 weeks gestational age with good fetal heart tones. Skin examination was notable for plaque-type psoriasis affecting approximately 40% of the patient's total body surface area. The plaques showed severe erythema, as well as moderate induration, scale, and pruritus. The most severely affected sites were the lower back, chest, abdomen, calves, and thighs. The disease had spared the patient's face, soles of her feet, and palms.

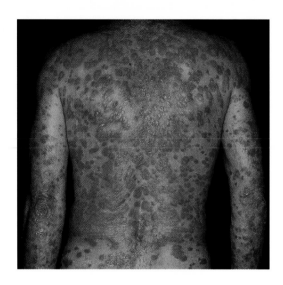

$\mathcal{Q}$uestion

$\mathcal{W}$hat is the safest management approach for a pregnant patient with wide-spread psoriasis?

$\mathcal{D}$iscussion

Although psoriasis tends to improve during pregnancy, it can worsen, with or without an associated traumatic event or, in a minority of cases, infection. Traditional Goeckerman therapy, conducted either in a hospital or a day treatment setting, is probably the safest treatment for widespread psoriasis in pregnant patients for whom topical therapies are neither effective nor feasible. Goeckerman or Ingram therapy, or the combination of the two, has been used for decades without evidence of significant harm to a pregnant woman or her fetus. UVB phototherapy is one of the safest treatment options available; theoretically, it is as safe as sunlight.

Excessive use of any topical corticosteroid should be avoided during pregnancy because of possible risk for adrenal suppression or Cushing's syndrome. Limited usage is considered safe. Studies among women given systemic corticosteroids during pregnancy have not found a related increase in birth defects.

PUVA therapy is generally not recommended during pregnancy even though studies have not found the therapy to increase birth defects significantly. The studies have not distinguished between bath PUVA or oral PUVA, however. Minimal or undetectable psoralen levels in the serum may develop after bath or topical "paint" PUVA therapy; thus, theoretically, the topical formulation is safer than systemic PUVA during pregnancy. Absolute safety of PUVA therapy has not been proved; such therapy may be an option if Goeckerman or Ingram therapy is not available.

Among the systemic agents, cyclosporine may pose the least risks to pregnant patients with severe psoriasis. In a recent study among 160 pregnant women receiving cyclosporine, there was no increase in birth defects. In contrast, methotrexate is associated with fetal demise; doses as low as 2.5 to 5.0 mg daily have resulted in various birth defects.

Retinoids are associated with severe birth defects and must not be used during pregnancy. Acitretin, which is expected to receive FDA approval soon, has a much shorter half-life than etretinate. However, this medication can be converted to etretinate in women who consume alcohol. Exact guidelines with regard to the use of acitretin in pregnant women have not been established.

𝒞linical Pearls and Pitfalls

1. Goeckerman or Ingram therapy is probably the safest and most effective treatment for widespread psoriasis in pregnant patients.
2. When outpatient UVB therapy alone is not effective and Goeckerman or Ingram therapy is not available, PUVA therapy may be considered. Topical or bath PUVA should be safer than systemic therapy.
3. Data suggest that cyclosporine may be the safest oral medication with regard to risk for birth defects.

Suggested Readings

1. David M, Lowe NJ, Halder RM, Borok M. Serum 8-methoxypsoralen (8-MOP) concentrations after bathwater delivery of 8-MOP plus UVA. *J Am Acad Dermatol.* 1990;5(pt 1):931-932.

2. Gomez MI, Azana JM, Arranz I, Harto A, Ledo A. Plasma levels of 8-methoxypsoralen after bath-PUVA for psoriasis: Relationship to disease severity. *Br J Dermatol.* 1995;133(1):37-40.

3. Hallman CP, Koo JY, Omohundro C, Lee J. Plasma levels of 8-methoxypsoralen after topical paint PUVA on nonpalmoplantar psoriatic skin. *J Am Acad Dermatol.* 1994;2(pt 1):273-275.

4. Kozlowski RD, Steinbrunner JV, MacKenzie AH, Clough JD, Wilke WS, Segal AM. Outcome of first-trimester exposure to low-dose methotrexate in eight patients with rheumatic disease. *Am J Med.* 1990;88(6):589-592.

5. Managing psoriasis treatments and pregnancy. *National Psoriasis Foundation Bulletin.* 1996:27(1):8-9.

6. Ostensen M. The effect of pregnancy on ankylosing spondylitis, psoriatic arthritis, and juvenile rheumatoid arthritis. *Am J Reprod Immunol.* 1992;28(3-4):235-237.

7. Pham CT, Koo JY. Plasma levels of 8-methoxypsoralen after topical paint PUVA. *J Am Acad Dermatol.* 1993;3:460-466.

8. Selim MM, Hegi V. Pustular eruption of pregnancy treated with locally administered PUVA. *Arch Dermatol.* 1990;126(4):443-444.

9. Stern RS, Lang R. Outcomes of pregnancies among women and partners of men with a history of exposure to methoxsalen photochemotherapy (PUVA) for the treatment of psoriasis. *Arch Dermatol.* 1991;127(3):347-350.

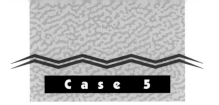
Chief Complaint

Hair loss

History of the Present Illness

A 7-year-old boy presented for a second opinion regarding his near total loss of scalp hair for 1 year. Topical steroids had failed to resolve the condition, and the boy had experienced only minimal regrowth following topical minoxidil therapy. He was otherwise in good health.

Physical Examination and Laboratory

Physical examination showed extensive nonscarring alopecia of the scalp and thinning of his eyebrows and eyelashes. There was hair on the boy's lower forehead and posterior neck.

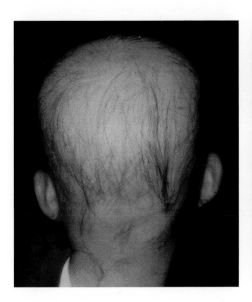
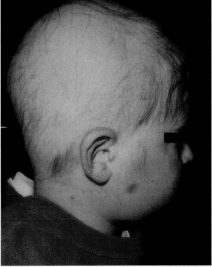

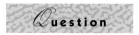

$\mathscr{W}$hat are the treatment options for severe alopecia areata?

$\mathscr{D}$iscussion

Therapies for severe alopecia areata include intralesional, topical, and systemic corticosteroids; contact irritants; contact allergens; PUVA; and topical minoxidil. These modalities may be used alone or in combination.

Intralesional corticosteroids are the gold standard of therapy for localized alopecia areata, but they offer limited benefit to patients with loss of more than 50% of scalp hair. The discomfort of intralesional injections can be ameliorated by pretreatment with EMLA. Ultrapotent and high-potency topical corticosteroids are often recommended for children with alopecia areata and can be used alone or in combination with topical minoxidil. Systemic corticosteroids are generally avoided in both adults and children with alopecia areata because of side effects as well as the risk for relapse of disease after discontinuation. Systemic corticosteroids have been reported beneficial in arresting and reversing rapidly progressive disease, however.

Anthralin (0.5%-1.0% cream), a contact irritant, may be utilized alone for localized or extensive disease in children and adults. Combination with topical minoxidil may be considered for adults with treatment-resistant disease. Adherence can be improved by gradually increasing the duration of daily applications or by applying the medication for up to 20 to 60 minutes on alternate days for the first 2 weeks of therapy. Patients and their parents need to be cautioned about staining of skin and fabric, folliculitis, and lymphadenopathy. Clinical irritation is not essential for clinical benefit. Cosmetically acceptable regrowth has been reported with anthralin alone or in combination with topical minoxidil.

Contact sensitizers, including dinitrochlorobenzene (DNCB), squaric acid dibutyl ester (SADBE), and diphenylcyclopropenone (DPCP), have been reported to achieve cosmetically acceptable hair growth in patients with severe alopecia areata. DNCB and SADBE are not commonly used because of mutagenic properties and instability in acetone, respectively. DPCP is advocated as monotherapy for adults with greater than 50% hair loss or for adults with treatment-resistant less extensive loss. Although sensitizers have been studied in children, a conservative approach is to avoid topical sensitization in this age group. Dermatitis, pruritus, blistering, and lymphadenopathy have been associated with topical sensitizers.

Topical and oral PUVA have been reported to exert variable efficacy in the treatment of alopecia areata. Recent retrospective evaluation showed limited value of PUVA therapy.

Topical minoxidil, particularly at 5% rather than the commercially available 2% concentration, may achieve cosmetically acceptable hair growth. Response is greater for patients with patchy loss affecting less than 75% of the scalp than for patients with more severe disease. Efficacy can be enhanced by use in combination with anthralin or ultrapotent topical steroids. Patients with alopecia totalis show little response to minoxidil alone or in combination. Mild hypertrichosis may affect areas beyond the scalp due to spread of minoxidil from the hands, dripping from the scalp onto the face, or from contact with the pillowcase. Minoxidil should be applied at least 1 hour before bedtime. The hypertrichosis should resolve with discontinuance of the drug.

𝒞linical Pearls and Pitfalls

1. Intralesional corticosteroids remain the gold standard for the treatment of localized alopecia areata.

2. Anthralin is recommended for the treatment of more widespread disease in children and adults. Topical minoxidil, alone or in combination with anthralin or topical steroids, is especially beneficial for hair loss affecting less than 75% of the scalp in children and adults. Topical sensitizers should be considered for adults with extensive or treatment-resistant disease.

3. Staining of the skin and fabrics, unwanted hypertrichosis, and dermatitis are adverse reactions associated with anthralin, topical minoxidil, and topical sensitization therapy, respectively.

Suggested Readings

1. Fiedler VC. Alopecia areata. A review of therapy, efficacy, safety, and mechanism. *Arch Dermatol.* 1992;128:1519-1529.
2. Shapiro J. Alopecia areata. Update on therapy. *Dermatol Clin.* 1993;11:35-46.
3. Shapiro J. Topical immunotherapy in the treatment of chronic severe alopecia areata. *Dermatol Clin.* 1993;11:611-617.
4. Taylor CR, Hawk JLM. PUVA treatment of alopecia areata partialis, totalis and universalis: Audit of 10 years' experience at St. John's Institute of Dermatology. *Br J Dermatol.* 1995;133:914-918.

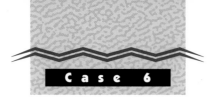

*C*ase 6

*C*hief Complaint

Generalized plaque psoriasis unresponsive to treatment with tar,
topical steroids, and antibiotics

*H*istory of the Present Illness

A 7-year-old girl presented at the psoriasis center with generalized plaque psoriasis. She had experienced a relentless flare of generalized plaque psoriasis for 3 months despite the use of 10% liquor carbonis detergens (LCD) in Aquaphor®, 0.1% triamcinolone acetonide (TAC) ointment, and various topical corticosteroids. The patient's family noted that sunlight seemed to make her psoriasis much worse. Her medical history was significant for asthma with one previous hospitalization. Her current medications included a bronchodilator inhaler. Both her brother and paternal grandfather had a history of psoriasis.

*P*hysical Examination

Examination revealed large plaque-type psoriasis of the lower extremities and the trunk. Diffuse involvement of the face and arms almost resembled erythroderma (Figs 1-3). Diffuse scalp involvement also was evident.

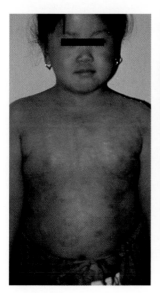 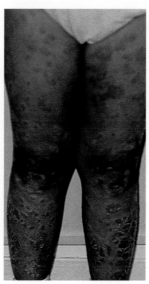 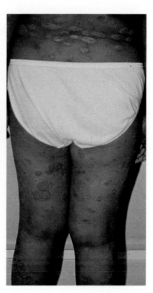

Figs 1-3 *Psoriasis extending over the anterior trunk, face, anterior thighs and calves, and posterior back, arms, and legs (day 1 of treatment).*

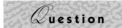

Question

*W*hat is the safest and most effective way to treat generalized, photosensitive plaque-type psoriasis unresponsive to outpatient topical medications in a 7-year-old?

Discussion

Photosensitive psoriasis is rare. The prevalence among psoriasis patients is estimated to be 5.5% in the adult population. The exact prevalence in the pediatric population is not known. In general, photosensitive psoriasis has a statistically higher frequency in patients with:

• Skin type I;
• A history of hereditary photosensitivity;
• Advanced age; and
• Psoriasis affecting the hands.

Polymorphous light eruption (PMLE) develops in one half of the patients with photosensitive psoriasis. In the remaining patients, the condition develops slowly following exposure to light.

Goeckerman therapy, conducted intensively in a day treatment setting or inpatient unit, poses the least risk for many patients, including those with acquired immunodeficiency syndrome (AIDS), pregnant patients, pediatric patients, and those with multiple medical problems. Black tar and phototherapy work by locally immunosuppressing the skin only; major side effects are limited to burning or irritation of the skin. There is little potential for damage to end organs via absorption of drug.

In this case of photosensitive psoriasis, UVB phototherapy worsened the patient's condition. Modified Goeckerman therapy was conducted at the Psoriasis Treatment Center without the use of UVB. In outpatient phototherapy, it is generally understood that UVB is the predominant therapeutic agent, while over-the-counter (OTC) tar preparations play a minor, adjunctive role in the treatment of psoriasis. The efficacy of tar is enhanced by the use of original black tar rather than LCD or other forms of OTC-diluted preparations (Figs 4, 5).

Rather than risk irritation of the intensely inflamed area with the use of black tar, the psoriasis was initially treated with 0.1% TAC ointment, applied several times daily, and 5% LCD in Nutraderm® for the scalp. As the erythroderma steadily decreased in intensity, the patient showed no adverse reaction to the use of 5% LCD, so the concentration of the scalp preparation was increased to 10% LCD in Nutraderm. Eventually, TAC ointment was decreased to 0.025%, and 2% crude coal tar (so-called black tar) was applied without adverse effects. The concentration of black tar was eventually increased to 10% crude coal tar with 2% salicylic acid, during which time, the use of TAC ointment was gradually discontinued. When the patient finished her treatment program after approximately 40 sessions, the psoriasis was more than 98% cleared (Fig 6).

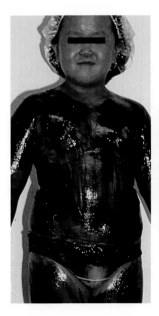 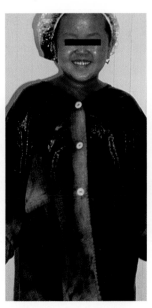 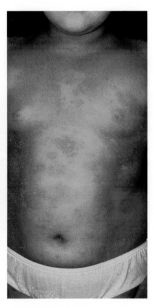

Fig 4 The patient's body was covered with 5% crude coal tar.

Fig 5 Note the patient's tar-soaked pajamas, which enhance treatment by providing an occlusive effect (treatment day 15).

Fig 6 Modified Goeckerman technique—increasing concentrations of daily black tar but no phototherapy, which could have worsened the skin condition—is effective: Lesions are flat; only postinflammatory hyperpigmentation remains.

$\mathscr{C}$linical Pearls and Pitfalls

1. Modified Goeckerman therapy—without the use of UVB—may be effective treatment for photosensitive psoriasis.

2. Patients generally do very well with black tar therapy without the concurrent use of phototherapy, in contrast to outpatient experience with OTC tar preparations that generally are not very effective without the concurrent use of UVB phototherapy.

3. Goeckerman therapy remains the safest alternative treatment for photosensitive psoriasis.

Suggested Readings

1. Morison WL. Phototherapy and photochemotherapy. *Adv Dermatol.* 1992;7:255-270.
2. Ros AM. Photosensitive psoriasis. *Sem Dermatol.* 1992;4:267-268.

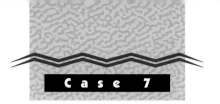

Case 7

Chief Complaint

Nonhealing facial lesions

History of the Present Illness

A 35-year-old woman with human immunodeficiency virus (HIV) infection was referred by the emergency department for a 5-week history of eruptive facial lesions. A biopsy performed 2 weeks earlier by another physician was consistent with pyogenic granuloma. There was no response to dicloxacillin sodium. The patient had not sought medical care for acquired immunodeficiency syndrome.

Physical Examination and Laboratory

Physical examination revealed multiple crusted papules and ulcerated red nodules affecting the central face. Telangiectasias were noted at the margins of several of the lesions. Repeat biopsy and review of the original biopsy showed a vascular proliferation characterized by plump endothelial cells with hyperchromatic nuclei and mitoses. A dense neutrophilic infiltrate was present. Clumps of organisms were apparent on routine histology and silver stain.

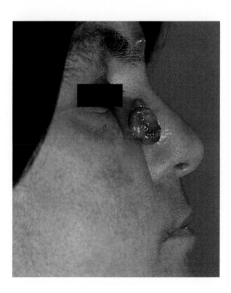

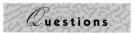

Questions

*W*hat are the diagnosis and differential diagnosis?

*W*hat are the potential systemic manifestations of this disease?

*W*hat other clinical syndromes are associated with the causative organism?

Discussion

Bacillary angiomatosis was first described in 1982 in one patient with subcutaneous nodules and fever and next in 1987 in several patients with HIV infection and multiple red papules and nodules. Recently there have been reports of bacillary angiomatosis in immunocompetent hosts.

The lesions of bacillary angiomatosis are most commonly misdiagnosed as Kaposi's sarcoma or pyogenic granulomas. Bacillary angiomatosis can be clinically and histologically distinguished from Kaposi's sarcoma. The lesions of bacillary angiomatosis at presentation are typically papules or nodules, usually blanch, tend to bleed, often are eruptive in size and number, and respond to antibiotics. The lesions of Kaposi's sarcoma are initially macules, patches, or plaques, often follow skin cleavage planes, rarely blanch or bleed, usually progress slowly, and do not respond to antibiotics. Histologically, the lesions of bacillary angiomatosis show sharp demarcation, lobular capillary proliferation, plump endothelial cells, many neutrophils, and granular clumps of bacteria. The lesions of Kaposi's sarcoma are poorly demarcated with spindled endothelial cells; neutrophils and bacteria are absent.

Although bacillary angiomatosis is usually limited to the skin, systemic involvement can occur even in the absence of skin lesions. Lymph nodes, lung pleura, bronchial mucosa, bones, brain, liver, bone marrow, and spleen may be infected. Bacillary peliosis hepatitis, or hepatic infection showing blood-filled cysts, may develop with or without simultaneous cutaneous infection. Nausea, vomiting, diarrhea, fever, chills, hepatosplenomegaly, and response to antibiotic therapy are the major clinical features of bacillary peliosis hepatis.

Rochalimaea henselae and *Rochalimaea quintana* have been identified as causative agents of bacillary angiomatosis. *R henselae* also causes cat scratch disease; *R quintana* can induce trench fever. Many patients with bacillary angiomatosis report exposure to cats.

Bacillary angiomatosis responds to treatment with oral erythromycin (500 mg three times daily), as well as doxycycline, minocycline, tetracycline, chloramphenicol, trimethoprim-sulfamethoxazole, azithromycin, and ciprofloxacin. Treatment duration may be for weeks or months; repeat courses of therapy may be needed to treat relapses.

*C*linical Pearls and Pitfalls

1. Eruptive vascular papules and nodules in HIV-infected patients should suggest the diagnosis of bacillary angiomatosis.
2. Biopsy for routine histology and silver stain will distinguish bacillary angiomatosis from Kaposi's sarcoma and pyogenic granuloma.
3. The excellent response of bacillary angiomatosis to antibiotics further distinguishes the condition from Kaposi's sarcoma and pyogenic granulomas.

Suggested Readings

1. Adal KA, Cockerell CJ, Petri WA. Cat scratch disease, bacillary angiomatosis, and other infections due to *Rochalimaea*. *N Engl J Med*. 1994;330:1509-1515.
2. Cockerell CJ. Bacillary angiomatosis and related diseases caused by *Rochalimaea*. *J Am Acad Dermatol*. 1995;32:783-790.
3. Cotell SL, Noskin GA. Bacillary angiomatosis. Clinical and histologic features, diagnosis, and treatment. *Arch Intern Med*. 1994;154:524-528.

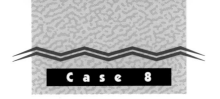

$\mathscr{C}$hief Complaint

Generalized severe plaque-type psoriasis

$\mathscr{H}$istory of the Present Illness

A 44-year-old Filipino-American male with a 15-year history of psoriasis and psoriatic arthritis presented at the Clinic seeking more effective therapy. In the past, he had used topical and systemic corticosteroids, methotrexate, etretinate, and hydroxyurea—all without lasting benefit. Also, he reported having tachyphylaxis related to the prior use of topical and systemic steroids. He discontinued methotrexate because of abnormalities in liver function tests as well as an abnormal liver biopsy. Moreover, at the time the abnormal liver biopsy was performed, methotrexate had become ineffective both for arthritis and psoriasis even at doses as high as 12 tablets per week. Etretinate failed to produce any therapeutic benefit, and the patient experienced serious xerosis as a side effect of the medication. Hydroxyurea was also totally ineffective despite the use of maximum doses.

$\mathscr{P}$hysical Examination

Physical evaluation revealed widespread involvement of plaque-type psoriasis affecting 80% of the patient's total body surface area, including the scalp, face, trunk, and all extremities (Fig 1).

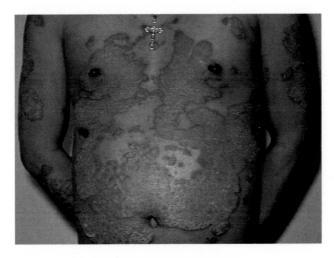

Fig 1 *Anterior trunk at patient presentation.*

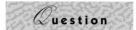

*W*hat new therapy is available for patients with psoriasis that is resistant to standard treatment?

Discussion

A new formulation of cyclosporine (Neoral®), which has received Food and Drug Administration approval, is available for use in patients undergoing transplantation. Even though it is well accepted that cyclosporine is often dramatically effective in the treatment of generalized psoriasis, one of the major difficulties with the use of the traditional agents is the wide variation in bioavailability. The broad interindividual differences in bioavailability, ranging from 10% to 90%, occur because cyclosporine needs to be "digested" with appropriate amounts of bile and pancreatic enzymes before it can be absorbed efficiently into the intestine. The absorption of cyclosporine takes place primarily in the small intestine. The efficiency of absorption can fluctuate extensively, depending on the availability of bile and pancreatic enzymes. Absorption does not take place until the intestinal content reaches the ampulla of Vater where bile and pancreatic juice flow into the lumen of the duodenum. In contrast, the new formulation is "predigested" and does not depend on interaction with bile and pancreatic enzymes for its absorption.

The patient received the new formulation of cyclosporine, beginning with a maximum dose of 5 mg/kg/d for the plaque-type psoriasis that affected 80% of total body surface area (Figs 2, 3). During the first 3 months of the 6-month treatment period, the patient's psoriasis cleared completely. He also had complete remission of severe psoriatic arthritis and joint pain, which had affected primarily the left third and fourth metatarsal joints and, when severe, would cause the patient to walk with a limp.

The exact dosage range for treatment of psoriasis with the new cyclosporine formulation has not been defined, but it may be less than the dosage that is required for traditional cyclosporine therapy.

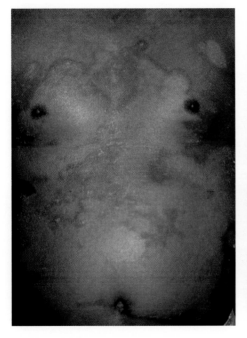

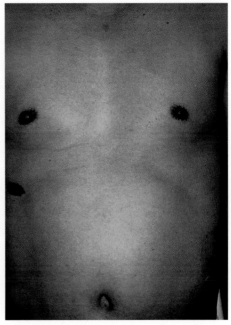

Fig 2 Therapeutic effects of new cyclosporine formulation at 2 weeks.

Fig 3 Therapeutic effects of new cyclosporine formulation at 6 weeks.

Clinical Pearls and Pitfalls

1. Cyclosporine may offer dramatic results for patients with generalized psoriasis, even if other treatments modalities, such as methotrexate, hydroxyurea, etretinate, and phototherapy, fail to improve the psoriasis.
2. A new cyclosporine formulation is absorbed more reliably and efficiently than the traditional formulation.
3. The bioavailability of the new cyclosporine formulation is enhanced because it is not dependent on bile and pancreatic enzyme interaction for absorption.
4. Dosage and treatment guidelines for the new formulation have not yet been established.

Suggested Readings

1. Drewe D, Beglinger C, Thoma A. The absorption site of cyclosporin in the human gastrointestinal tract. *Clin Pharmacol.* 1992;33:39-43.
2. Drewe J, Meier R, Vonderscher J, et al. Enhancement of the oral absorption of cyclosporin in man. *Br J Clin Pharmacol.* 1992;34(1):60-64.
3. Holt DW, Mueller EA, Koverik JM, van Bree JB, Kutz K. The pharmacokinetics of Sandimmun Neoral: A new oral formulation of cyclosporin. *Transplant Proceed.* 1994;26(5):2935-2939.
4. Kovarik JM, Mueller EA, van Bree JB, Tetzloff W, et al. Reduced inter- and intraindividual variability in cyclosporin pharmacokinetics from a microemulsion formulation. *J Pharm Sci.* 1994;83(3):444-446.
5. Vonderscher J, Meinzer A. Rationale for the development of Sandimmun Neoral. *Transplant Proceed.* 1994;26(5):2925-2937.

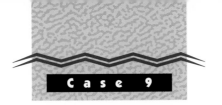

Chief Complaint

Sores on the lips, tongue, and left cheek

History of the Present Illness

A 50-year-old woman with no significant medical history presented with an acneform eruption on her left cheek of 3 weeks' duration. The left cheek subsequently became crusted and shortly thereafter she developed "cold sores" on her lips and tongue. She has only been able to eat soft foods for the past 10 days. She also noted a new lesion between the fingers. She had received treatment from her family physician for bacterial infection.

Physical Examination and Laboratory

Examination revealed thickly crusted erosions affecting both lips, erosions with pseudomembranous exudate affecting the tongue, and grouped crusted erosions on the left cheek and left nose. One vesicle was noted in a web space of the hand. After obtaining negative cultures for herpesvirus and the patient's failure to respond to oral acyclovir, biopsies of an erosion from the cheek and perilesional skin were performed. Routine histologic analysis demonstrated an intraepidermal vesicle with suprabasilar acantholysis. Direct immunofluorescence showed deposition of IgG and C3 in the epidermal intercellular spaces. A diagnosis of pemphigus vulgaris was made.

Although the cutaneous lesions responded to high-dose oral corticosteroids, the oral lesions failed to respond. Repeat cultures from lip samples for herpesvirus were positive. The patient experienced dramatic improvement with intravenous (IV) corticosteroids and IV acyclovir. The patient continues to do well with tapering doses of prednisone, azathioprine 50 mg twice a day, and acyclovir 400 mg twice daily.

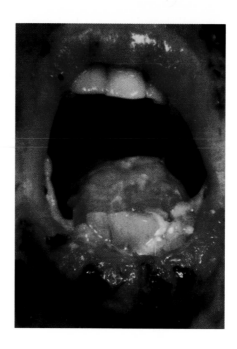

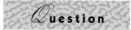

$\mathcal{Q}$uestion

$\mathcal{W}$hat is the clinical differential diagnosis?

$\mathcal{D}$iscussion

The leading clinical diagnostic considerations in this case were herpetic gingivostomatitis with whitlow, herpes simplex virus (HSV) infection with erythema multiforme, and pemphigus complicated by HSV infection.

Primary herpetic gingivostomatitis typically affects children, adolescents, and young adults. Primary infection may be clinically silent or may be full blown with extensive, painful vesicles and erosions of the tongue, gingiva, palate, buccal mucosa, and lips. Fever, malaise, lymphadenopathy, and sore throat often accompany severe primary infection. Herpetic whitlow may complicate primary mucosal infection.

While nearly all cases of erythema multiforme minor are thought to be linked to HSV, erythema multiforme major is more often due to drugs. Buccal erosions and blisters with cervical lymphadenopathy may be seen in erythema multiforme minor, while the buccal mucosa, vermilion, palate, gingiva, and tongue are typically affected in erythema multiforme major.

Oral disease is invariable in pemphigus vulgaris and usually is the first manifestation of the disease. The buccal mucosa is most commonly affected, but the mucosal involvement can extend from the vermilion to the distal esophagus. Paraneoplastic pemphigus is also characterized by oral disease affecting the vermilion, gingival, buccal, and lingual mucosa.

Pemphigus can be complicated by HSV infection of the oral mucosa, as was the case with this patient. Concomitant HSV infection should be considered when a pemphigus patient with stable disease has an acute worsening of oral involvement.

Clinical Pearls and Pitfalls

1. Painful erosions of the tongue, lip, palate, and buccal mucosa may accompany primary herpetic gingivostomatitis, erythema multiforme major, pemphigus vulgaris, and paraneoplastic pemphigus.
2. Biopsy and culture are important in establishing an accurate diagnosis and in directing treatment.
3. HSV infection can complicate pemphigus vulgaris and should be considered when pemphigus patients have acute exacerbations of oral disease.

Suggested Readings

1. Balciunas BA, Kelly M, Siegel MA. Clinical management of common oral lesions. *Cutis*. 1991;47:31-36.
2. Mutasim DF, Pelc NJ, Anhalt GJ. Paraneoplastic pemphigus. *Dermatol Clin*. 1993;11:473-481.
3. Prendiville JS, Israel DM, Wood WS, et al. Oral pemphigus vulgaris associated with inflammatory bowel disease and herpetic gingivostomatitis in an 11-year-old girl. *Pediatr Dermatol*. 1994;11:145-150.
4. Siegel MA, Balciunas BA, Kelly M, et al. Diagnosis and management of commonly occurring oral vesiculoerosive disorders. *Cutis*. 1991;47:39-43.

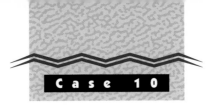

Chief Complaint

Nonhealing ulcers of the ears

History of the Present Illness

A 38-year-old man was referred for evaluation and management of multiple nonhealing, painful ulcers of the anterior and posterior surfaces of the ears. The ulcers had started developing 9 months earlier. The patient had not experienced any improvement despite treatment with numerous oral and topical antibiotics and prednisone (40 mg daily). The patient was otherwise in good health, and review of systems was negative for diabetes mellitus, arthritis, bowel disease, and sinus or nasal symptoms. He complained of a cyst preauricularly, which had been biopsied recently; the patient noted that the biopsy site seemed to be enlarging.

Physical Examination and Laboratory

Deep ulcers with prominent eschar affected the anterior and posterior surfaces of the ears, sparing the ear lobes. An early ulcer was present preauricularly. The nasal septum was intact. Biopsy of the preauricular lesion showed granulomatous dermatitis without vasculitis; special stains and cultures were negative for microorganisms. Results from tests assessing rheumatoid factor, serum protein electrophoresis, chest radiography, antineutrophil cytoplasmic autoantibody (ANCA), and renal function were normal. The patient responded to one course of pulse methylprednisolone with complete resolution of the ulcers affecting the ears. The preauricular ulceration also improved, but ultimately chronic dapsone therapy and intermittent intralesional corticosteroid therapy were required to treat the ulcer.

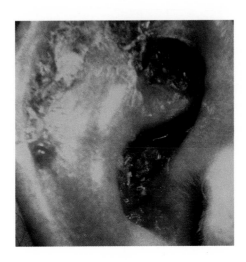

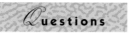

*W*hat is the differential diagnosis?

*W*hat systemic conditions are associated with this disease?

*D*iscussion

After infectious etiologies were excluded, the leading diagnostic considerations in this case were inflammatory dermatoses, including relapsing polychondritis, Wegener's granulomatosis, and pyoderma gangrenosum.

Relapsing polychondritis is characterized by auricular and nasal chondritis. The cartilaginous aspects of the external ears show episodic erythema, warmth, and edema that spare the ear lobe and eventuate in fibrosis. Arthritis, ocular inflammation, and respiratory chondritis are also common.

Wegener's granulomatosis is a systemic vasculitis that affects the upper and lower respiratory tract and kidney, as well as other organ systems, including the skin and oral mucosa. Granulomatous inflammation of the respiratory tract may lead to sinusitis, destruction of the cartilage of the nasal septum with saddle nose deformity, and pulmonary nodules with cavitation. The kidneys commonly develop glomerulonephritis. Although mucocutaneous lesions can precede systemic involvement, generally mucocutaneous disease is indicative of active systemic disease, especially that affecting the joints and kidneys. Dermatologic manifestations include palpable purpura, oral, genital, and cutaneous ulcers, nodules, pustules, and livedo reticularis. The level of ANCA correlates with disease activity.

Pyoderma gangrenosum is considered a diagnosis of exclusion, made only after biopsy for histology and culture, as well as examination of other organ systems exclude conditions such as infection, vasculitis, malignancy, and peripheral vascular disease. Pyoderma gangrenosum usually begins as a pustule on an erythematous or dusky base, which rapidly evolves into an undermined, serpiginous ulcer with a violaceous border and purulent base. Ulcers may develop in response to trauma and heal with a cribriform pattern. The legs are most commonly affected, although truncal involvement is not infrequent. Pyoderma gangrenosum of the head and neck, which was previously considered a distinct disease termed malignant pyoderma, is relatively rare. The disease shows a predilection for the periauricular region.

Diseases associated with pyoderma gangrenosum include inflammatory bowel disease, rheumatoid arthritis, benign monoclonal gammopathy (especially IgA), and lymphoproliferative malignancies. It has also been described in association with Wegener's granulomatosis and relapsing polychondritis; however, in as many as 50% of cases, pyoderma gangrenosum is unrelated to systemic disease.

Clinical Pearls and Pitfalls

1. Pyoderma gangrenosum is a diagnosis made after conditions including infections, vasculitis, malignancy, and peripheral vascular disease are excluded.
2. Rarely, pyoderma gangrenosum may affect the head and neck with a predilection for periauricular areas.

Suggested Readings

1. Duguid CM, Powell FC. Pyoderma gangrenosum. *Clin Dermatol.* 1993;11:129-133.
2. Frances C, Du LT, Piette JC, et al. Wegener's granulomatosis. Dermatological manifestations in 75 cases with clinicopathologic correlation. *Arch Dermatol.* 1994;130:861-867.
3. Hedayati H, Zuzga JJ Jr, Faber DB. Rheumatoid arthritis, relapsing polychondritis, and pyoderma gangrenosum evolving into non-Hodgkin's lymphoma. *J Am Osteopath Assoc.* 1993;93:240-242, 246-248.
4. Schwaegerle SM, Bergfeld WF, Senitzer D, et al. Pyoderma gangrenosum: A review. *J Am Acad Dermatol.* 1988;18:559-568.
5. Wernikoff S, Merritt C, Briggaman RA, et al. Malignant pyoderma or pyoderma gangrenosum of the head and neck? *Arch Dermatol.* 1987;123:371-375.

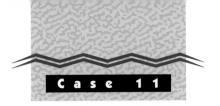

*C*hief Complaint

Severe hand and foot pustular psoriasis as well as severe plaque-type psoriasis

*H*istory of the Present Illness

A 41-year-old black female presented with a 2-year history of severe hand and foot pustular psoriasis, as well as severe plaque psoriasis. The patient's medical history was significant for hypertension. She also had a history of chronic hepatitis C infection, which had developed secondary to "crack" cocaine abuse.

Because of the patient's medical history, she was not eligible for many of the therapies for severe recalcitrant psoriasis. She could not take methotrexate because of her history of chronic hepatitis C infection. The patient was not a candidate for etretinate because she was of childbearing age. She could not take cyclosporine because she had a history of severe hypertension and borderline renal function tests.

The patient was admitted to the Psoriasis Day Treatment Center, where she received treatment for 5 weeks. After 25 days of topical treatment, localized quartz light treatments, Burow's soaks, UVB phototherapy, and 5% crude coal tar applied to the plaques (but not the pustular areas), the psoriasis improved significantly, clearing in up to 95% of the afflicted sites. Treatment with isotretinoin was attempted during the Day Treatment Program, and in a supervised setting, the patient was able to take medication at a dosage of 60 mg/d for approximately a 2-week period. This greatly facilitated clearance of the pustular psoriasis on her feet and lower calves. Near the end of the treatment stay, however, the patient complained of severe headaches. Because of this, isotretinoin was discontinued.

The patient continued outpatient UVB phototherapy and the use of refined tar as an outpatient for several weeks, but eventually, pustular psoriasis recurred. Within 2 months, the patient returned to the Psoriasis Treatment Center with a severe flare-up of pustular and plaque psoriasis.

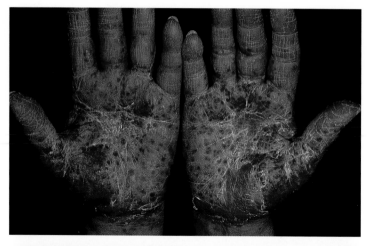

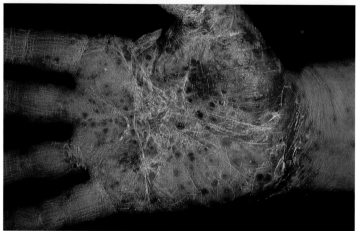

Question

$\mathcal{W}$hat treatment option is still available for this case of recalcitrant, pustular psoriasis?

Discussion

Treatment options that are still available include PUVA phototherapy, 6-thioguanine (6-TG), and hydroxyurea. When the patient was discharged from the Day Treatment Program, she was not able to return on a regular basis for PUVA therapy; thus, this option was not feasible. Between the options of using hydroxyurea or 6-TG, hydroxyurea was chosen first because it has less tendency to cause a precipitous drop in the hematocrit. Although hydroxyurea is not approved for treatment of psoriasis, it turned out to be very effective for this patient.

Baseline laboratory measures were obtained, and the drug was started at a dosage of 500 mg twice daily. The patient's complete blood cell (CBC) count was monitored approximately every 2 weeks. After the first 2 weeks of initiation of hydroxyurea treatment, the patient's plaque psoriasis was noted to be significantly flatter than on her previous visits. The dose was increased to 500 mg three times a day. On the patient's next visit 2 weeks later, the psoriasis continued to show significant improvement and flattening. The patient reported no side effects. The CBC count remained stable, and there was no change in the platelet count or liver function.

Some published literature regarding the use of hydroxyurea for psoriasis gives an impression that one almost has to induce mild anemia before clinical improvement in the psoriasis occurs. Hydroxyurea appears to be a very safe medication, which can be used long term in various dosages. The usual dosage for adults is 500 mg twice daily. If necessary, the dosage can be increased to 500 mg three times a day. Anemia is a rare complication; however, almost every patient eventually develops macrocytosis. If macrocytosis does not lead to macrocytic anemia, it is of no clinical consequence. To minimize the chance of developing anemia, patients are routinely given folic acid (1 mg twice daily) to be taken with hydroxyurea.

Because hydroxyurea is not as reliably effective as etretinate or methotrexate, it is most often used in combination with UVB or PUVA therapy. Photosensitivity from hydroxyurea has not been observed in our experience.

$\mathscr{C}$linical Pearls and Pitfalls

1. Hydroxyurea can be a safe and effective alternative for patients who fail most other treatment options. Although hydroxyurea is not as reliably effective as methotrexate or some other more frequently used medications, for those patients who respond to it, it can be a safer alternative to other medications.

2. Hydroxyurea is generally not hepatotoxic. No liver biopsies are required even if hydroxyurea is used chronically.

3. Almost every patient receiving long-term hydroxyurea treatment develops macrocytosis. It is of no clinical consequence as long as the patient does not develop macrocytic anemia. Patients are given folic acid to minimize the risk of developing anemia.

Suggested Readings

1. Baker H. Psoriasis. In: Farber EM, Cox AJ, eds. *Proceedings of the 33rd International Symposium*. New York: Grune & Stratton; 1982:119.

2. Layton AM, Sheehan-Dare RA, Goodfield MJD, Cotterill JA. Hydroxyurea in the management of therapy resistant psoriasis. *Br J Dermatol*. 1989;121:647-653.

3. Moschella SL, Greenwald MA. Psoriasis with hydroxyurea. An 18-month study of 60 patients. *Arch Dermatol*. 1973;107:363.

4. Wright S, Baker H. Hydroxyurea. In: Roenigk HH, Maibach HI, eds. *Psoriasis*. 2nd ed. New York: Marcel Dekker; 1991:577-581.

5. Yarbro JW. Hydroxyurea in the treatment of refractory psoriasis. *Lancet*. 1969; 18:846-847.

6. Yarbro JW, Leavell UW Jr. Refractory psoriasis—a new approach to the management. *IM J Ill Med*. 1971;139:152-154.

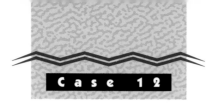
Chief Complaint

Thick and yellow nails

History of the Present Illness

A 45-year-old marketing executive complained of a 5-year history of thick and yellow nails that affected his hands and feet. He had a long history of tinea pedis and occasionally had required treatment for the condition. A 15-month course of griseofulvin failed to improve the condition of the patient's toenails but did clear the fingernail condition; however, the fingernail dystrophia returned following discontinuance of the medication. The patient's medical history was otherwise unremarkable, except for allergic rhinitis, for which he had received terfenadine intermittently. The patient was very motivated to treat his nails because the fingernail involvement caused him embarrassment when meeting with business clients.

Physical Examination and Laboratory

Examination revealed scaling of both soles, toe webs, and the right palm. Three fingernails of each hand and all nails of the feet were dystrophic, showing varying degrees of onycholysis, yellow discoloration, and subungual debris. The crural area was clear. Potassium hydroxide (KOH) preparation from the palm and toe webs demonstrated hyphal elements. Fungal cultures from nail samples were negative, but periodic acid-Schiff (PAS) staining of nail plates demonstrated hyphal elements.

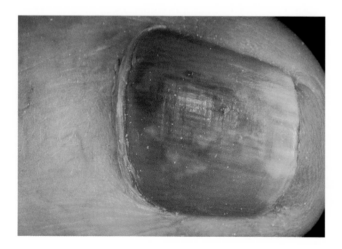

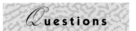

Questions

*W*hat diagnostic techniques are utilized to confirm the clinical diagnosis of onychomycosis?

*W*hat are the advantages and risks of new systemic agents for the treatment of onychomycosis?

Discussion

Ideally, the clinical diagnosis of onychomycosis should be confirmed prior to initiating systemic therapy. Fungal culture and KOH preparation are the most commonly used confirmatory tests. Fungal cultures may yield false-positive results when nonpathogenic contaminants are isolated. False-negative culture results may be due to sampling technique (fungi from distal nail samples may be dead) and/or choice of culture medium. KOH preparation from thick nail debris can be difficult to interpret; stains can be added to help outline the fungal walls.

Histopathologic examination of nail plate clippings with PAS staining augments culture and KOH testing; dermatophytes, yeasts, and molds may show distinctive features on routine histopathologic examination, although the specific pathogen is not identified. Immunohistochemistry and flow cytometry are experimental techniques that permit more precise determination of causative organisms when cultures are negative or when cultures isolate multiple organisms. Greater diagnostic specificity may be important in guiding treatment.

Until recently, griseofulvin and ketoconazole were the only oral therapies available for the treatment of onychomycosis. Both require prolonged daily courses of treatment, have a low cure rate for pedal nail disease, and are associated with a high relapse rate. Griseofulvin is effective only against dermatophytes; ketoconazole is a broad-spectrum agent, but it carries the risk for idiosyncratic hepatotoxicity.

Fluconazole, a broad-spectrum antimicrobial agent, has been successfully prescribed for the treatment of onychomycosis in a pulse fashion, 150 mg one dose per week for 9 months. The medication is rarely associated with hepatotoxicity.

Itraconazole and terbinafine are incorporated into the nail plate rapidly and persist there for prolonged periods. Both medications can be administered for relatively brief periods—daily for 3 months for toenails and for 6 weeks for fingernails—or in a pulse fashion. Patients should be advised that although the duration of treatment is short, the nail will not appear clinically normal until it grows out over a 6- to 9-month period for fingernails and over a 12- to 18-month period for toenails.

Itraconazole and terbinafine are clinically much more effective than griseofulvin and ketoconazole, especially for the treatment of toenail disease, although treatment failures and relapses may occur. Itraconazole is a broad-spectrum fungistatic agent, while terbinafine has in vitro fungicidal activity against dermatophytes, *Scopulariopsis,* and *Candida parapsilosis* and fungistatic activity against *Candida albicans.*

Gastrointestinal disturbances and rashes are the most common adverse reactions to itraconazole and terbinafine. The risk for hepatotoxicity with itraconazole therapy appears to be very low, but liver functions tests should be conducted during treatment. Rarely, terbinafine has been associated with hematologic abnormalities. Taste disturbances, including a metallic taste, affect fewer than 1% of patients receiving the medication. These effects are reversible 2 to 5 weeks after discontinuance of the drug. Itraconazole should be taken with food, while terbinafine is well absorbed regardless of food intake. Itraconazole interacts with numerous medications, and a careful medication history must be obtained before initiating therapy; life-threatening arrhythmias can ensue with concomitant astemizole, terfenadine, or cisapride, and severe hypoglycemia can occur with concomitant oral hypoglycemic therapy. Drug interactions are much less common with terbinafine, though rifampin may increase its clearance, while cimetidine may decrease it. The dose of terbinafine should be halved in patients with creatinine clearance less than 50 mL/min. Patients who are allergic to other azole medications may be allergic to itraconazole. Both itraconazole and terbinafine are contraindicated during pregnancy and in nursing mothers.

*C*linical Pearls and Pitfalls

1. Fungal cultures of nails can yield false-negative and false-positive results. Histopathologic examination of the nail plate can complement culture results and can help confirm the clinical diagnosis of onychomycosis. Immunohistochemistry and flow cytometry are experimental techniques that may be routinely used to diagnose onychomycosis in the future.

2. Although itraconazole and terbinafine have excellent safety profiles, patients should be fully informed of the risks of therapy. The potential for significant drug interactions should be addressed with any patient considering itraconazole treatment.

3. Patients should be aware that although the duration of treatment with itraconazole and terbinafine is short, there will be a lag time before the nail plate grows out completely and clinical cure is evident.

Suggested Readings

1. Elewski BE. Onychomycosis. *Fitzpatrick's J Clin Dermatol.* 1994;2:48-54.
2. Pierard GE, Arrese JE, De Doncker P, et al. Present and potential diagnostic techniques in onychomycosis. *J Am Acad Dermatol.* 1996;34:273-277.
3. Shear NH, Gupta AK. Terbinafine for the treatment of pedal onychomycosis: A foot closer to the promised land of cured nails? *Arch Dermatol.* 1995;131:937-942.

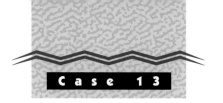

Chief Complaint

Habitual hair pulling

History of the Present Illness

A 27-year-old female with a history of hair-pulling since age 12 years reported that her hair pulling first started as a "nervous habit" and that she gave no thought to her action. However, repeated pulling on the hair resulted in patches of alopecia. The patient made a conscious effort to stop the hair-pulling activity at age 15 years and stated that she was able to prevent herself from pulling her hair from that time until she was age 20 years.

It seems that stresses in her life have precipitated the patient's pulling on her hair. She stated that she became more preoccupied with pulling her hair out when she turned 20 years old. At that point, she had graduated from high school and had a lot of free time. The hair-pulling activity became even worse after she married. She had a difficult relationship with her husband, which caused the patient to pull her hair out and pick at it for several hours a day. She would feel an overwhelming urge to pull at her hair, especially if she made a conscious effort to try to stop the activity. She felt as though she had to pull on her hair in order to release tension from the hair follicles; she reported feeling a brief relief after pulling out her hair, but that later, she would become very angry with herself for yielding to her destructive urges.

Physical Examination and Laboratory

Physical exam revealed a large central patch of self-induced alopecia over the parieto-occipital scalp (Fig 1). Scattered broken hair was observed in the area of the alopecia. The patient wore a hairpiece to cover the alopecia.

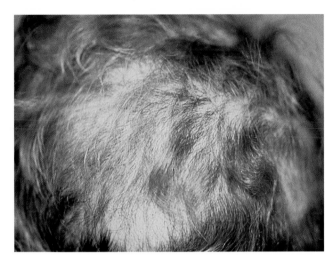

Fig 1 *Central areas of occipito-parietal alopecia with scattered broken hairs prior to patient receiving psychopharmacotherapy. A portion of the hairpiece the patient wore is visualized lateral to the alopecia.*

Question

What are effective treatment modalities for trichotillomania?

Discussion

Psychotherapy has traditionally been available for the treatment of obsessive-compulsive disorders. However, clinical efficacy of psychotherapy has been unpredictable for this particular type of disorder. Behavioral therapy is thought to be more effective than other nonpharmacologic options; however, many psychodermatologic patients resist referrals to mental health professionals. In such cases, the use of medications may be the most feasible way for a dermatologist to try to treat these conditions.

There are three medications currently approved by the Food and Drug Administration for use in obsessive-compulsive disorders in the United States: clomipramine, fluoxetine, and fluvoxamine. Fluoxetine and fluvoxamine are somewhat easier to take than the tricyclic antidepressant clomipramine, which is associated with such adverse effects as sedation, orthostatic hypotension, weight gain, and anticholinergic side effects (dry mouth and constipation).

The initial assessment of the patient was that she was suffering from trichotillomania, with obsessive-compulsive disorder as the underlying cause for the behavior. She was given fluoxetine (20 mg/d). The patient began noticing improvement in her ability to focus on accomplishing daily tasks as well as a slightly easier time of stopping her compulsive pulling activity after approximately 2 months of treatment. At that time, she was taking low-dose fluoxetine with no side effects. The medication was increased to 40 mg/d. Approximately $1\frac{1}{2}$ months later, the patient reported even further improvement in her efforts to stop pulling her hair and picking her scalp and less preoccupation with the activity. She also felt somewhat less depressed. The fluoxetine dosage was increased to 60 mg/d. After 4 months of treatment, the patient noted significant improvement in her obsessive-compulsive tendencies. She spent a lot less time in front of the mirror pulling out her hair. In addition, she was much less depressed. Of note, part of this improvement may have been due to the fact that the patient had ended her relationship with her abusive spouse.

On physical examination, the patient had definite hair regrowth noted in previous patches of alopecia (Fig 2). Observation of her mental status revealed a more alert, smiling, coherent patient.

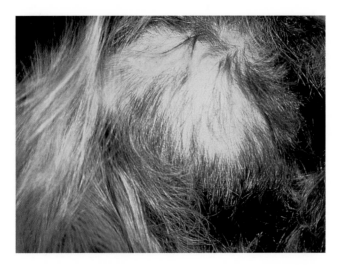

Fig 2 *After 6 months of psychopharmacotherapy, central hair regrowth is evident, reflective of diminished patient compulsion to pull her hair out.*

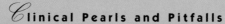

Clinical Pearls and Pitfalls

1. Trichotillomania can be successfully treated with psychotherapy or behavioral therapy, although psychotherapy has been less than reliable in terms of efficacy.

2. Three medications are approved for the treatment of obsessive-compulsive disorders in the United States.

3. When patients are started on antiobsessive-compulsive medications, they also need to be reminded that they must keep up their vigilance and motivation; these medications are not "magic bullets" that work entirely by themselves.

Suggested Readings

1. Koo JYM. Psychodermatology: A practical manual for clinicians. *Current Problems in Dermatology.* 1995;7(6):199-234.
2. Koo JYM, Pham CT. Psychodermatology: Practical guidelines on pharmacotherapy. *Arch Dermatol.* 1992;128:381-386.
3. Koo JYM: Psychotropic agents in dermatology. *Dermatol Clin.* 1993;11:215.

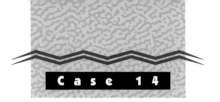

Chief Complaint

Worsening flexural dermatitis

History of the Present Illness

A 24-year-old woman with atopic dermatitis affecting the antecubital and popliteal fossae showed no improvement despite use of triamcinolone acetonide. She moisturizes twice daily and also occasionally uses triple antibiotic ointment for excoriated areas.

Physical Examination

Examination showed lichenified and excoriated plaques affecting the flexors. Patch testing was positive to lanolin, neomycin, and budesonide.

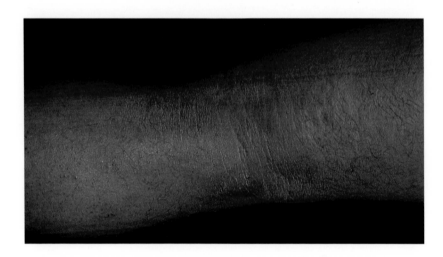

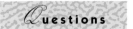

$\mathscr{Q}$uestions

$\mathscr{W}$hich patients are at risk for corticosteroid contact allergy?

$\mathscr{W}$hat are the best test reagents for corticosteroid contact allergy?

$\mathscr{W}$hat advice should be given to patients with corticosteroid contact allergy?

$\mathscr{D}$iscussion

Delayed-type hypersensitivity reactions may occur to vehicles and preservatives present in commercial corticosteroid preparations, as well as to the corticosteroid itself. Corticosteroid contact allergy is becoming increasingly recognized, affecting 2% to 5% of patients evaluated in contact dermatitis centers. Corticosteroid contact allergy more often affects patients with stasis dermatitis, chronic actinic dermatitis, perineal dermatitis, treatment-resistant dermatitis, and multiple medicament sensitivities.

Patch testing for corticosteroid contact allergy is complicated by controversy regarding optimal screening agents, optimal test concentration and vehicles, and cross-reaction patterns.

Tixocortol and budesonide, which are available in Europe and Canada but not in the United States as standardized patch test allergens, are considered excellent screens for corticosteroid contact allergy. Budesonide is now available in the United States as an inhaler, and patch testing may be performed to the aerosolized agent. Testing to hydrocortisone 17-butyrate and alclometasone dipropionate also may be helpful for identifying patients with corticosteroid contact allergy; both are available as commercial topical corticosteroid preparations in the United States.

Cross reaction has been reported to occur more frequently within four groups of structurally related corticosteroids, but exceptions to this scheme have been observed; therefore, recommendations for allergen substitution are difficult to make for the corticosteroid-sensitive patient. Patch testing or use testing to multiple commercially available corticosteroid creams and ointments should be performed to determine which products may be used safely. Finally, interpreting patch test reactions can be difficult because of corticosteroid-induced vascular constriction effects; allergic reactions are best detected at delayed readings between days 4 and 6.

Rarely, patients with corticosteroid contact allergy have been observed to develop generalized cutaneous reactions with the administration of systemic corticosteroids. Therefore, only those corticosteroids to which the patient has responded negatively on patch testing should be administered systemically.

$\mathcal{C}$linical Pearls and Pitfalls

1. Delayed-type hypersensitivity reactions can occur to vehicles and preservatives present in commercial topical corticosteroid products and to the corticosteroid itself.
2. Tixocortol and budesonide are the preferred screens for corticosteroid contact allergy but are not routinely available as standardized reagents in the United States.
3. When standardized allergens are not available, patch testing may be performed to commercially available budesonide inhaler, topical hydrocortisone 17-butyrate, and topical alclometasone dipropionate.
4. Patients with corticosteroid contact allergy should undergo testing to commercial topical steroid creams and ointments to identify those that are safe for use.

Suggested Readings

1. Dooms-Goosens A. Corticosteroid contact allergy: A challenge to patch testing. *Am J Contact Dermatitis.* 1993;4:120-122.
2. Rietschel RL. Patch testing for corticosteroid allergy in the United States. *Arch Dermatol.* 1995;131:91-92.
3. Wilkinson SM. Hypersensitivity to topical corticosteroids. *Clin Exp Dermatol.* 1994;19:1-11.

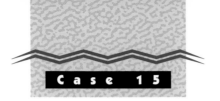

Chief Complaint

Persistent uremic pruritus

History of the Present Illness

A 47-year-old woman with a history of uremic pruritus presented at the Psoriasis Treatment Center after having tried numerous pharmacologic therapies, including doxepin hydrochloride (HCl), hydroxyzine HCl, and diphenhydramine HCl, often at very high doses, without any symptomatic relief of her pruritus. Indeed, the pruritus was so severe that the patient was hospitalized several times for secondary cellulitis as a result of excoriation.

Physical Examination

The patient was noted to have generalized excoriations on the trunk and all extremities. She had patches of eczema on her extremities, but the area of involvement with pruritus extended far beyond the confines of patchy eczema.

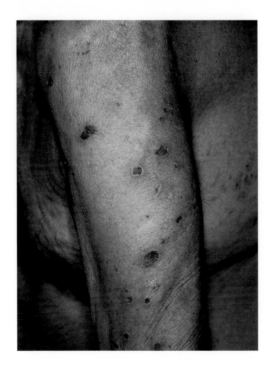

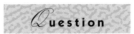
Question

Is phototherapy effective for the treatment of uremic pruritus?

Discussion

UVB phototherapy is known to be one of the most effective and safest treatments for uremic pruritus. Unfortunately, up to 90% of patients with chronic renal failure experience significant problems with uremic pruritus from time to time, and many of these patients never receive phototherapy. This is frequently due to a lack of interaction between the nephrologist and the dermatologist who has phototherapy equipment. One of the best ways to facilitate referrals from dialysis centers to help control this prevalent problem is to present the efficacy of UVB phototherapy for the treatment of uremic pruritus not only to the nephrology attendings but also to the nursing staff and other professionals in dialysis clinics.

The patient began receiving UVB phototherapy at the Psoriasis Treatment Center. After undergoing phototherapy 2 to 3 times weekly for several months, her generalized pruritus improved significantly and eventually resolved. When she experienced recurrence of pruritus weeks or months later, she would restart UVB phototherapy with a similar response, usually within 3 to 4 weeks. By undergoing outpatient UVB phototherapy—a dose of UVB light applied to the total body and maintained at approximately 200 millijoules—the patient has remained essentially itch-free for the last 2½ years. She notes that if she misses her phototherapy treatment for any significant duration of time during those periods when she requires retreatment, the pruritus tends to worsen. She also uses topical corticosteroids on eczema-type patches as well as various moisturizers to prevent xerosis.

Uremic pruritus is associated with chronic renal failure in patients undergoing hemodialysis. Serum histamine levels have been shown to be elevated in chronic renal failure patients with pruritus, and UVB therapy has been reported to be beneficial for the relief of pruritus in these patients. There is evidence that UVB radiation is able to suppress histamine release from mast cells. In one study, the sera of chronic renal failure patients with uremic pruritus was found to contain some histamine-releasing factors, which can be depleted or diminished by UVB radiation. The details of how this occurs on a cellular level, however, remain unknown.

Another study showed that pre-UVB total plasma calcium level correlated directly with itching intensity but not with mast cell number. The study also showed that plasma phosphate levels were not statistically related to itching or mast cell number. In conclusion, it is not known whether hypercalcemia, in and of itself, or histamine release from mast cells is responsible for the severe itching these patients experience, but UVB phototherapy definitely provides symptomatic relief for cases in which other modalities such as topical or oral steroids have failed.

In more practical terms, treatment of uremic pruritus is generally conducted with UVB phototherapy applied three times per week. The general rules, such as a gradual increase in total light application and the importance of avoiding the burning threshold, apply to these cases as well as to treatment of psoriasis or eczema with UVB phototherapy. It generally takes several weeks for the pruritus to respond. Once resolved, the pruritus usually remains in remission for several months.

𝒞linical Pearls and Pitfalls

1. Uremic pruritus occurs frequently among patients receiving chronic dialysis therapy.
2. UVB phototherapy is one of the most effective and safest approaches to the treatment of uremic pruritus.
3. Generally, therapeutic response is observed over several weeks following initiation of phototherapy. The patient usually receives intermittent treatment as symptoms recur.

Suggested Readings

1. Cohen EP, Russell TJ, Garancis JC. Mast cells and calcium in severe uremic itching. *Am J Med Sci.*1992;303(6):360-365.
2. Imazu LE, Tachibana T, Danno K, Tanaka M, Imamura S. Histamine-releasing factor(s) in sera of uraemic pruritus patients in a possible mechanism of UVB therapy. *Arch Dermatol Res. (Archiv fur Dermatologische Forschung.)* 1993;285(7):423-427.
3. Tan JK, Haberman HF, Coldman AJ. Identifying effective treatments for uremic pruritus. *J Am Acad Dermatol.* 1991;Nov, 25(5 Pt 1):811-818.

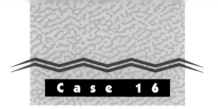

*C*hief Complaint

Stinging, itching, and hives from latex gloves

*H*istory of the Present Illness

A 30-year-old nurse with a history of flexural dermatitis and allergic rhinitis complained of stinging, itching, and hives within 30 minutes of donning latex gloves. Two years earlier she had developed hand dermatitis, which improved over the weekends, gradually worsened during the course of the work week, and was responsive to topical steroid therapy. Radioallergosorbent testing (RAST) was positive for latex antibodies. Patch testing showed positive reactions to thiuram and carba mix.

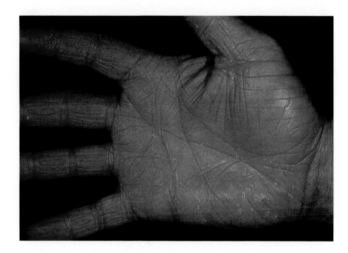

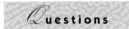

Questions

*W*hat types of reactions do health care workers develop to rubber latex gloves?

*W*hat groups are at risk for latex allergy?

*H*ow is latex allergy diagnosed?

*W*hat advice should be given to patients with latex allergy?

Discussion

Reactions to rubber latex gloves include irritant contact dermatitis, immediate hypersensitivity reactions, and delayed-type hypersensitivity reactions. Irritant contact dermatitis in health care workers may be due to sweating under gloves, frequent hand-washing, and glove powder. Immediate hypersensitivity reactions ranging from contact urticaria, allergic rhinitis, asthma, and anaphylaxis are due to IgE-mediated reactions to the latex protein. The latex antigen can become trapped in the glove powder and aerosolized when latex gloves are donned or removed.

Delayed-type hypersensitivity reactions or allergic contact dermatitis are most often secondary to accelerators—thiuram, carba, mercaptobenzothiazole—added to latex in the manufacturing process. Affected health care workers generally show a gradual progression over a period of years from hand dermatitis to contact urticaria to respiratory signs and symptoms to anaphylaxis. Health care workers who are allergic to latex also may demonstrate delayed hypersensitivity to allergens, including rubber accelerators that speed the process of glove manufacture.

Immediate hypersensitivity reactions to latex were first reported in 1979. A sharp increase in latex allergy was reported in the late 1980s following institution of universal precautions and after the production of poorly manufactured, highly allergenic gloves.

The prevalence of latex allergy in health care workers is approximately 8% and as high as 24% in atopic workers. Prevalence among patients with spina bifida and those with urogenital anomalies that require frequent bladder catheterization and multiple surgeries has been reported to range from 30% to nearly 70%. Individuals who are allergic to kiwi, banana, avocado, or chestnut also may be allergic to latex.

Latex allergy can be diagnosed by RAST, skin testing, or use testing. RAST identifies only approximately 50% of latex-allergic persons. Skin testing can be hazardous; resuscitation equipment should be available. The risk for anaphylaxis during skin testing can be decreased by making a single prick, rather than multiple pricks, and by pricking superficially. Neither RAST nor skin testing to latex is standardized at this time. The use test entails wearing part or all of the latex glove on wet skin for 20 minutes and observing it for contact urticaria.

Latex-allergic individuals should avoid latex medical devices, latex products in the home, and cross-reacting fruits. Prophylaxis with systemic corticosteroids and antihistamines prior to medical procedures has been unsuccessful. Persons who have experienced systemic signs and symptoms of latex allergy should wear bracelets that alert others to their condition. Health care workers who have an asymptomatic RAST response or those who have a positive prick test and negative use test may wear low-protein latex gloves for work but should not have mucosal exposure to latex when undergoing medical or surgical procedures.

$\mathcal{C}$linical Pearls and Pitfalls

1. Reactions to latex rubber gloves include irritant dermatitis, IgE-mediated hypersensitivity, and allergic contact dermatitis.
2. Patients with spina bifida, atopic health care professionals, and individuals allergic to kiwi, banana, avocado, or chestnut are at high risk for latex allergy.
3. Prophylaxis prior to latex exposure has been unsuccessful. Rather, careful avoidance of latex-containing medical devices, home products, and cross-reacting foods is essential for the latex-allergic individual.

Suggested Readings

1. Hamann CP. Natural rubber latex protein sensitivity in review. *Am J Contact Dermatitis.* 1993;4:4-21.
2. Sussman GL, Beezhold DH. Allergy to latex rubber. *Ann Intern Med.* 1995;122:43-46.
3. Taylor JS, Praditsuwan P. Latex allergy: Review of 44 cases including outcome and frequent association with allergic hand eczema. *Arch Dermatol.* 1996;132:265-271.

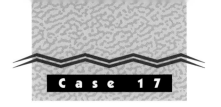

*C*hief Complaint

Chronic pruritus, formication, and delusions of parasitosis

*H*istory of the Present Illness

A 44-year-old Caucasian man with chronic pruritus and formication (tactile hallucination involving the belief that something is crawling on the body or under the skin) described intense itching accompanied by crawling, biting and stinging sensations. He felt these sensations all over the body. The patient also described a "parasite," which he had seen on his skin. This parasite, according to the patient, was a round insect with two antennae, black to red in color, and moved on his skin with its legs. As he detailed, this insect crawled from the patient's skin into the hair follicles. When it tried to get back onto the skin, the patient's abnormal skin sensations were localized to the scalp, face, chest, groin, shins, and feet. Instead of scratching to rid himself of the parasite, the patient had tried a number of topical agents to kill the "bug."

The patient self-treated himself with various medications, including Kwell® lotion, Elimite® cream, over-the-counter anti-infestation agents, sulfasalazine, metronidazole, Phisoderm®, Malathion®, Ivermectin® (dog heartworm medicine), Vermox®, prednisone, haloperidol, doxepin HCl, and, finally, pimozide. The patient reported that none of the medications really helped him that much, although he noted that after he stopped pimozide (2 mg/d), the formication symptoms worsened. The patient had initially been given pimozide by his primary dermatologist. He discontinued the treatment because he thought he was experiencing some sedative effect from the medication, even though he was only taking 1 tablet per day. Besides mild sedation, the patient did not recall any serious side effects. He reported that even though he was not heavily sedated, he had to do his work as a high school teacher, and he was not able to function well at work while taking pimozide.

The family history is of some interest. The patient stated that his father-in-law and other members of the family had also developed similar symptoms. This reinforced his belief that he was infested with some type of parasite. The patient said that the symptoms began after he helped his brother-in-law and sister-in-law fix their septic tank. He believed that he contracted the bugs from his parents-in-law and sister-in-law who were present at that time. Eventually, his wife had the same problem, but she was able to rid herself of the parasites with Elimite cream. In fact, during his consultation, the patient brought in his father-in-law, who clearly believed that both he and the patient were infested with some type of parasite. The patient's extended family lived in New Mexico, rural California, and Utah. Several members of the patient's family from these three locations complained of the same infestation symptoms; yet, physicians throughout the Southwest had failed to resolve or diagnose their conditions.

The patient was so concerned about his infestation, and at the same time, very concerned that his primary dermatologist did not believe that he had a real infestation that he challenged his dermatologist to switch socks with him for 24 hours. The patient believed that the dermatologist would then acquire the infestation within a matter of hours. The dermatologist did switch socks with the patient but did not acquire any evidence of infestation. On close questioning, the patient stated that the first symptom he had experienced was intense pruritus. Eventually, other perceptions such as crawling and biting sensations became associated with the pruritus. It was at this time that the patient began to think that the pruritus was due to some infestation with parasites.

Physical Examination

Physical examination revealed no clinical evidence of infestation or any other primary skin disorder.

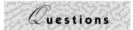

Questions

How do the patient's sensory complaints relate to his delusional ideation?

What is folie à deux?

What is the treatment of choice for delusional parasitosis?

Discussion

This case illustrates two important aspects of dealing with some cases of delusions of parasitosis. The first point is that for some patients with delusions of parasitosis, it is not only important to try to treat the delusion with pimozide, but it may also be therapeutic to try to eradicate the sensory complaint, which in fact may be the primary pathology in some patients with delusions of parasitosis. Although there are rare patients with delusions of parasitosis who only have the delusion without any cutaneous symptoms, most patients also experience formication (crawling and biting sensations) and/or intense pruritus.

It has been speculated that some, if not most, of these patients for whom a sensory complaint precedes the development of a delusional belief system, the delusion may actually be a way for the patient to explain what he or she felt on the skin. In this particular case, it is impossible to know how much of the patient's clinical improvement was due to the therapeutic effect of pimozide or to the control of his pruritus with the Goeckerman regimen, which he received after discontinuing the pimozide therapy. When managing patients with delusions of parasitosis, every possible therapeutic channel must be explored: Controlling the primary skin sensation is one of the more important aspects of treatment.

Secondly, this case illustrates the importance of working with these patients pragmatically. Having this patient receive therapy with the Goeckerman regimen was not only helpful in controlling his primary sensation of pruritus, but also removed him from his work and family environments. Removing the patient from his family helped break up the *folie à deux* situation. In such a situation, usually one of the individuals is dominant and the other is passively going along with the dominant person's delusional system. In this particular case, the patient, himself, was the dominant character in terms of having an active delusional ideation. However, if this patient had been the passive one, simply the fact that he was removed from the dominant one in his family could have led to the clinical improvement.

The treatment of choice for delusional parasitosis is the antipsychotic medication pimozide. Pimozide is known to be much more efficacious than other antipsychotic medications for the treatment of delusional parasitosis, perhaps due to its unique effectiveness in diminishing or eliminating formication. Pimozide is not only a dopamine-blocking agent, but also a potent opiate receptor-blocking agent. This pharmacologic effect of pimozide in blocking opiate receptors is thought to be responsible for its efficacy in diminishing both formication and pruritus. The dosage of pimozide can be started as low as 1 mg/d ($\frac{1}{2}$ tablet) and increased by 1 mg every week until the desired effect is obtained. Significantly decreased formication and dramatically lower mental preoccupation regarding infestation are achieved in most patients at a dosage of 4 to 6 mg/d (2 to 3 tablets daily).

At these very low doses, cardiac side effects are extremely unusual. However, it is still recommended that pretreatment electrocardiography (ECG) be obtained and repeated when a dosage of two to three tablets daily is reached. Diphenhydramine HCl, 25 mg as needed four times a day for stiffness or restlessness, is usually prescribed in case the patient experiences pseudo-Parkinsonian side effects. For many patients, pimozide can be used episodically; once the symptoms are under control, the therapeutically effective dose is maintained for 1 to 2 months and then gradually tapered, thus minimizing the risk for long-term side effects.

*C*linical Pearls and Pitfalls

1. Sensory complaints may be the primary pathology underlying delusional ideation.
2. Pimozide is the pharmacologic treatment of choice for treatment of delusional parasitosis.

Suggested Readings

1. Koo JYM. Psychodermatology: A practical manual for clinicians. *Current Problems in Dermatology.* 1995;7;199-234.
2. Koo JYM: Psychotropic agents in dermatology. *Dermatol Clin.* 1993;11:215.
3. Koo JYM. Skin Disorder. Psychogenic factors affecting medical conditions. In: *Comprehensive Textbook of Psychiatry.* 1995;26(7):1928-1929.
4. Damiani JT, Flowers FP, Pierce DK. Pimozide in delusions of parasitosis. *J Am Acad Dermatol.* 1990;Feb:212-213.

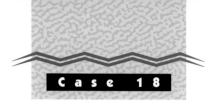

Case 18

*C*hief Complaint

Itchy rash of the vulva (red-to-white plaque)

*H*istory of the Present Illness

A 55-year-old woman complained of a 6-month history of an itchy rash of the vulva, which had failed to respond to topical steroids, topical and oral antifungal therapy, and antihistamines. Her medical history was unremarkable, and a recent pelvic examination was normal except for the vulvar rash.

*P*hysical Examination and Laboratory

Examination showed well-demarcated red plaques with mild scaling and crusting affecting the labia majora. There were no satellite lesions. The nails, nasolabial folds, elbows, knees, inframammary areas, axillae, umbilicus, and scalp were clear. Potassium hydroxide (KOH) preparation was negative. Biopsy revealed single cells within the epidermis and nest of cells with large pleomorphic nuclei and abundant pale-staining cytoplasm. Focally, some of the clusters of cells showed a central lumen. Periodic acid Schiff (PAS) testing was positive for these "Paget" cells; they were also diastase-resistant, colloidal-iron stain positive and Alcian blue positive at pH 2.5. Immunohistochemically, these cells were S100 negative and positive for carcinoembryonic antigen.

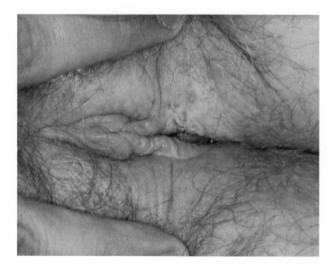

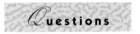
Questions

*W*hat is the diagnosis?

*W*hat conditions may be associated with this disease?

Discussion

Extramammary Paget's disease is a rare disorder characterized by well-demarcated red plaques affecting regions rich in apocrine glands, including the vulva, penis, scrotum, perianal area, and axillae. Extramammary Paget's disease affecting apocrine poor sites, such as the back, buttocks, and lower chest, has been reported less commonly. Simultaneous involvement of the axillary and anogenital regions has been described.

Clinically, extramammary Paget's disease may be confused with psoriasis, seborrheic dermatitis, candidiasis, contact dermatitis, and squamous cell carcinoma. Failure to respond to treatment for inflammatory dermatoses and absence of associated stigmata—for example, nail pitting or scalp disease suggestive of psoriasis—should prompt biopsy. Histologically, extramammary Paget's disease should be distinguished from melanoma and Bowen's disease.

Patients with extramammary Paget's disease are at increased risk for associated malignancies. A review of 197 cases reported over a 20-year period found that 12% of patients have an associated concurrent underlying malignancy, the location of which is usually closely related to the location of the cutaneous lesion. Perianal extramammary Paget's disease is associated with adenocarcinoma of the gastrointestinal tract, while penile, scrotal, groin, and vulvar diseases are associated with adenocarcinoma of the genitourinary tract. Vulvar extramammary Paget's disease is also associated with breast cancer.

Extramammary Paget's disease is associated with an underlying cutaneous adnexal carcinoma in nearly one fourth of patients. Adenocarcinoma arises in the epidermis and then locally invades adnexal structures. Subsequent dermal extension can lead to metastatic disease.

Treatment of disease localized to the skin is generally surgical excision, including the Mohs' technique; radiation and chemotherapy are alternatives for patients who are poor surgical candidates.

Clinical Pearls and Pitfalls

1. Extramammary Paget's disease should be considered in the differential diagnosis of red plaques affecting apocrine-rich sites.
2. Inadequate response to therapy for a presumed inflammatory or infectious dermatosis in an apocrine-rich site should prompt early biopsy.
3. Patients with extramammary Paget's disease should be evaluated for underlying malignancy of the gastrointestinal tract, genitourinary system, and breast.

Suggested Readings

1. Chanda JJ. Extramammary Paget's disease: Prognosis and relationship to internal malignancy. *J Am Acad Dermatol.* 1985;13:1009-1014.
2. Hemann WR. Extramammary Paget's disease. *Clin Dermatol.* 1993;11:83-87.

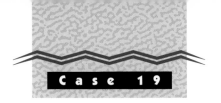

Chief Complaint

Red, scaly primary lesion with development of similar lesions at various sites

History of the Present Illness

A 72-year-old Caucasian man with insulin-dependent diabetes mellitus, hypertriglyceridemia, and hypertension presented with a 40-year history of a red, scaly lesion on his left upper inner thigh. The patient described the appearance of similar lesions on his right thigh, neck, and left buttock within the past 6 months. He denied pruritus, oral lesions, and a family history of similar lesions. The patient had applied triamcinolone acetonide 0.025% ointment twice daily for 2 weeks without improvement. His other medications included gemfibrozil, metoprolol tartrate and hydrochlorothiazide, and insulin. The patient stated that he had no known allergies to any medications.

Physical Examination and Laboratory

Potassium hydroxide (KOH) testing and fungal culture of samples from the lesions were negative. Biopsy of the left thigh lesion showed a focal, vertical tier of parakeratosis and scattered dyskeratotic cells underlying this area. The lesions were diagnosed as porokeratosis of Mibelli.

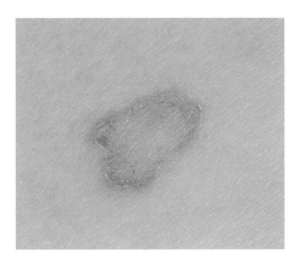

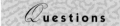

Questions

*W*hat conditions are included in the differential diagnosis of porokeratosis of Mibelli?

*W*hat are the primary concerns associated with this condition?

*W*hat are the treatment options for porokeratosis of Mibelli?

Discussion

Porokeratosis of Mibelli is one of five types of primary porokeratosis specifically characterized by a few prominent hyperkeratotic and verrucous lesions that can develop in different areas of the skin and mucous membranes. A chronic condition of hereditary origin, porokeratosis of Mibelli typically appears as one or several keratotic papules on the hands, feet and legs, face, scalp, buccal mucosa, and perineal region. The disease emerges when the patient is young and progresses very slowly over time. It affects twice as many males as females.

Porokeratosis of Mibelli is distinguished clinically from four other variants of porokeratosis. Disseminated superficial actinic porokeratosis (DSAP) usually manifests itself as several lesions on sun-exposed areas of skin during the third or fourth decade. Porokeratosis palmaris et plantaris disseminata (PPPD), occurring during the second or third decade, consists of more numerous lesions beginning on the palms and soles and later spreading to both sun-exposed and nonexposed skin. A rare form of porokeratosis, called punctate porokeratosis, is limited to the palms and soles and consists of more punctate, keratotic, spinelike lesions. Linear porokeratosis—characterized by several lesions in a linear or zosteriform distribution—is the fifth clinical variant.

The primary concerns with this chronic condition are accurate diagnosis and monitoring for malignant transformation. Porokeratosis of Mibelli is typically confused with lichen planus, actinic keratosis, tinea infection, verrucae, lichen sclerosus, and epithelial nevi. Cutaneous T-cell lymphoma may resemble the disease. Histologic examination, showing hyperkeratosis, parakeratosis, and acanthosis in the epidermis with a classic cornoid lamella (column of parakeratotic nuclei and keratin extending from the stratum corneum into an absent granular cell layer), is most specific. Changes in the dermis are minimal but may demonstrate a mild inflammatory infiltrate and decreased adnexal structures, such as hair follicles and sebaceous glands.

Lesions of porokeratosis may undergo malignant transformation, particularly when in a linear distribution. It is therefore important to make an accurate diagnosis and set up appropriate follow-up appointments for the patient. Cultured fibroblasts from patients with porokeratosis of Mibelli have demonstrated chromosomal instability. One series of patients had squamous cell carcinoma, Bowen's disease, or basal cell carcinoma develop within the lesions of porokeratosis. As many as 7.5% of cutaneous malignancies (squamous cell carcinoma, Bowen's disease, or basal cell carcinoma) may arise within these lesions. Patients of advanced age with long-standing lesions and those with larger lesions on the extremities in a linear distribution are at highest risk for malignant transformation.

Eradication of porokeratosis lesions, either surgically or medically when possible, would appear to be significant due to their increased tendency toward malignant transformation. For smaller lesions, cryotherapy, excision, or carbon dioxide laser ablation are viable options. For widespread lesions, direct application of 5-fluorouracil solution, with or without occlusion, has been used. Both etretinate and isotretinoin have shown temporary effectiveness, but recurrence of the lesions is common after discontinuance of therapy. In cases of disseminated porokeratosis of Mibelli, more conservative measures may be warranted. Additionally, patients should receive education on self-examination and the proper use of sunscreens.

Clinical Pearls and Pitfalls

1. Porokeratosis of Mibelli may mimic other treatable dermatologic conditions, and thus, must be distinguished from these. Histologic examination is the most specific diagnostic tool.
2. Porokeratosis lesions may undergo malignant transformation, frequently developing into squamous cell carcinoma or basal cell carcinoma.
3. Proper monitoring of lesions and avoidance of sun exposure are important measures to manage porokeratosis of Mibelli.

Suggested Readings

1. Chernosky ME. Porokeratosis. *Arch Dermatol.* 1986;122:869.
2. Breneman DL, Breneman JC. Cutaneous T-cell lymphoma mimicking porokeratosis of Mibelli. *J Am Acad Dermatol.* 1993;20:1046-1048.
3. McDonald SG. Porokeratosis (Mibelli). *J Am Acad Dermatol.* 1983;8:107.
4. Taylor AMR, Harnden DG, Fairburn EA. Chromosomal instability associated with susceptibility to malignant disease in patients with porokeratosis of Mibelli. *J Natl Cancer Inst.* 1973;51:371-376.
5. James WD. Squamous cell carcinoma arising in porokeratosis of Mibelli. *Int J Dermatol.* 1986;25:389.
6. Sasson M, Krain AD. Porokeratosis and cutaneous malignancy: A review. *Dermatol Surg.* 1996;22:339-342.
7. Lozinski AZ. Metastatic squamous cell carcinoma in linear porokeratosis of Mibelli. *J Am Acad Dermatol.* 1987;16:448.
8. Campbell JP. Disseminated superficial actinic porokeratosis. *Int J Dermatol.* 1985;24:261.

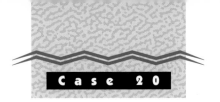

*C*hief Complaint

Nonhealing red rash on the penis

*H*istory of the Present Illness

A 60-year-old man presented with a persistent rash on the penis that failed to improve with topical steroid and antifungal therapies. He was a widower and was no longer sexually active. His medical history was remarkable only for diabetes mellitus that he was able to control with diet.

*P*hysical Examination and Laboratory

The examination was significant for a velvety, shiny, red thin plaque on the glans. The patient was uncircumcised. There was no significant inguinal lymphadenopathy. Fungal culture was negative. Biopsy revealed atypical epithelial hyperplasia involving all the cell layers of the epithelium. The atypical keratinocytes demonstrated large hyperchromatic and pleomorphic nuclei and eosinophilic cytoplasm. The underlying stroma was chronically inflamed.

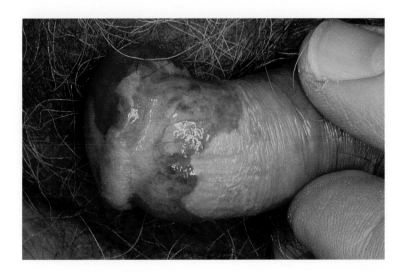

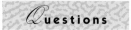

Questions

*W*hat is the diagnosis?

*W*hat are the treatment options?

Discussion

Erythroplasia of Queyrat, or squamous cell carcinoma in situ, is characterized by single or multiple red, velvety, glistening atrophic plaques affecting the glans, urethral meatus, frenulum, corona, sulcus, or prepuce. Ulceration or verrucous changes may be indicative of more invasive disease. Erythroplasia of Queyrat primarily affects uncircumcised men. The average age at diagnosis is 50 years.

Erythroplasia of Queyrat must be distinguished from clinical mimics, such as psoriasis, candidal balanitis, plasma cell or Zoon's balanitis, contact dermatitis, erosive lichen planus, and fixed-drug reactions. Bowenoid papulosis is histologically indistinguishable from erythroplasia of Queyrat, but the clinical presentation differs. Bowenoid papulosis typically affects younger men, more often affects the shaft rather than the glans, is manifested by small papules that may coalesce to form plaques, and clinically may be confused with seborrheic keratoses and genital warts.

Generally, surgical excision is the recommended treatment for erythroplasia of Queyrat. When surgery is potentially disfiguring, other options include radiation therapy, topical 5-fluorouracil, and laser ablation. Mohs' micrographic surgery should be considered for tissue conservation. Circumcision is considered beneficial to prevent local recurrence.

Clinical Pearls and Pitfalls

1. Erythroplasia of Queyrat should be considered in the differential diagnosis of red plaques affecting the glans penis, along with inflammatory dermatoses, such as psoriasis, erosive lichen planus, fixed-drug reactions, and plasma cell balanitis, as well as candidal balanitis.

2. Failure of an erythematous plaque affecting the glans to respond to topical steroid or antifungal therapy should prompt biopsy to exclude malignancy.

Suggested Reading

1. Gerber GS. Carcinoma in situ of the penis. *J Urol.* 1994;151:829-833.

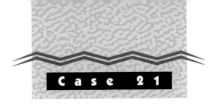

Chief Complaint

Widespread desquamation of skin on chest and arms following thalidomide therapy

History of the Present Illness

Acute lymphocytic leukemia was diagnosed in an 11-year-old male approximately 2 years before the patient presented at the Psoriasis Treatment Center. He had undergone bone marrow transplantation, and graft versus host disease (GVHD) developed about 4 months later. The patient was receiving several immunosuppressive medications as a result of his disease, including prednisone, acyclovir, cyclosporine, intravenous immune gammaglobulin, and azathioprine.

The patient developed the acute skin changes associated with GVHD. Initially, a mildly pruritic, blanchable, erythematous morbilliform eruption was the sole manifestation, but later it evolved into a lichenoid form of GVHD, characterized by violaceous, lichenoid papules on the distal aspects of the extremities, palms, and soles. In addition, large plaques of morpheaform sclerosis developed on his chest and back. The patient had been referred to the Center for PUVA treatment of the skin manifestations of GVHD. He underwent oral PUVA sessions three times weekly, for a total of 49 treatment sessions. Initially, the psoralen dose was 10 mg; it was gradually increased to 20 mg per treatment session. The patient first received 0.25 joules of UVA phototherapy, which was progressively increased to 7.5 joules of phototherapy to the total body, as well as 1 joule of UVB phototherapy to the face.

Because of the failure of the various immunosuppressive agents and the exacerbation of the disease, hematology services decided to initiate thalidomide therapy. Approximately 1 week after the initiation of thalidomide therapy, the patient experienced widespread desquamation of skin on his chest and arms.

Physical Examination

Physical examination, which took place soon after appearance of the thalidomide-induced rash, revealed erythematous, mildly scaly, inflammatory eczematoid eruptions covering more than 60% of the total body surfaces; the trunk and extremities were most intensely involved. A few days later, the intensity of the erythema subsided significantly, and areas of involvement exhibited diffuse desquamation.

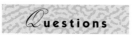

Questions

*W*hat is the likely etiology of this eruption?

*H*ow is graft versus host disease generally treated with respect to skin manifestations?

Discussion

The patient had experienced a very similar type of reaction when thalidomide therapy was attempted 1 year earlier. The rash during the previous episode apparently resolved following discontinuance of the thalidomide. Following outbreak of the second rash, the drug was once again discontinued.

PUVA therapy continued for 1½ weeks during which time the patient did not receive thalidomide. A skin biopsy performed at day 8 showed changes consistent with an acute drug eruption rather than acute exacerbation of GVHD. On day 10, the erythema and skin desquamation showed significant improvement.

GVHD, a frequent complication of bone marrow transplantation, is a clinical syndrome characterized by cutaneous changes, diarrhea, and liver dysfunction. There are two clinically distinguishable forms — acute and chronic. Both forms may have devastating cutaneous manifestations. The acute form, which usually develops 10 to 40 days after bone marrow transplantation, is associated with skin manifestations ranging from a mildly pruritic, blanchable, erythematous morbilliform eruption to full-thickness epidermal necrosis, which is indistinguishable from toxic epidermal necrolysis.

Chronic GVHD, which may occur months to years after bone marrow transplantation, may or may not be preceded by acute GVHD, and occurs in two forms. The first form is the lichenoid chronic GVHD, which is characterized by violaceous, lichenoid papules, commonly on the distal aspects of the extremities, palms, and soles. The second form, sclerodermoid GVHD, usually develops later and is characterized by plaques of sclerosis, which may resemble morphea and range in size from 1 to 10 cm. The disease also may be characterized by large confluent, sclerotic areas similar to scleroderma that cause significant discomfort, loss of mobility, and joint contractures.

The total number of PUVA treatments required to resolve lesions can range from 2 to 60; the average number of joules/cm^2 extend from 6.5 to 190. Patients can experience phototoxicity, sometimes requiring them to stop treatment, even when thalidomide is part of the treatment regimen. It is not clear whether other immunosuppressive agents such as cyclosporine, azathioprine, or prednisone change the response to phototherapy in any manner.

Several theories have been proposed as to how PUVA works to improve GVHD. PUVA therapy may clear cutaneous GVHD by suppressing the immune response that gives rise to this condition. One hypothesis that supports this on a cellular level is that most likely the PUVA treatment is selectively cytotoxic for activated lymphoid cells in the inflammatory infiltrate. Therefore, elimination of these cells results in cessation of damage to the epidermis and resolution of disease. Another hypothesis is that PUVA therapy may alter the target cells in the epidermis that provide the antigenic stimulation and/or mediators responsible for maintaining the immune response. Therapy with PUVA does damage keratinocytes and alter Langerhans' cells, which are potential target cells. A third theory is that PUVA therapy may induce an immune response to suppress GVHD. In this manner, PUVA therapy may suppress contact hypersensitivity. Also, PUVA therapy may induce a cell-mediated immune response by generation of antigen-specific T-suppressor cells.

Generally, in this setting, the patient initially receives PUVA treatment 3 to 4 times weekly. A preliminary course of four to six exposures may be useful if there are concerns about particular photosensitivity. Initial doses should be low because phototoxicity can develop unexpectedly. The reason for this is not clear but could be multifactorial and include the fact that hypopigmentation is often present, modulation of erythemal responses by these drugs often being employed as concurrent therapies, or photosensitivity due to the disease itself.

To assess treatment progress better and to avoid any rebound phenomenon the dosages of any immunosuppressive medication should remain constant until clearance of the disease. Improvement can be expected as early as the fifth treatment period, but an adequate trial of treatment should probably consist of 15 to 20 exposures. Once the lesions are resolved, weekly maintenance treatments should continue for up to 6 months. Finally, it is important to remember that PUVA therapy for GVHD is not a routine use of this modality, as it is with psoriasis and other diseases. The patients are often very sick, and fatal problems can develop rapidly and easily. Therefore, these patients require additional care and attention.

ℰlinical Pearls and Pitfalls

1. GVHD can be successfully treated with either thalidomide or PUVA therapy.
2. Drug eruption from thalidomide or any other acute, generalized inflammatory process can be exacerbated by PUVA phototherapy. While the patient is experiencing a widespread inflammatory process, especially resulting from a condition other than the original disease, PUVA therapy should be discontinued until the rash resolves.
3. A skin biopsy can be helpful in determining whether the sudden, unexpected skin eruption represents an exacerbation of GVHD or drug eruption.

Suggested Readings

1. Jampel RM, Farmer ER, Vogelsing GB, et. al. PUVA therapy for chronic cutaneous graft vs host disease. *Arch Dermatol.* 1991;127:1673-1678.
2. Vogelsgang GB, Farmer ER, Hess AP, et al. Thalidomide for the treatment of chronic graft vs host disease. *N Engl J Med.* 1992;326:1055-1058.

Chief Complaint

Blisters and scars on the hands

History of the Present Illness

A 16-year-old female presented with blistering and scarring of the dorsal hands and face. Her medical history was significant for juvenile rheumatoid arthritis that had been treated with naproxen sodium.

Physical Examination

Examination showed blisters, crusted erosions, and milia over the dorsal hands and erosions and scarring over the face. Biopsy of a vesicle of the dorsal hand revealed a noninflammatory subepidermal blister; direct immunofluorescence showed antibody deposition around blood vessels. Twenty-four hour urine and stool collections demonstrated normal levels of porphyrins.

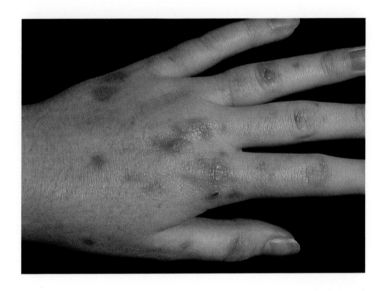

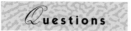

*W*hat is the diagnosis?

*W*hat drugs are associated with the condition?

*D*iscussion

The clinical manifestations of drug-induced pseudoporphyria mimic those of porphyria cutanea tarda (PCT), with blisters, skin fragility, scars, and milia over sun-exposed skin; sclerodermic changes and hirsutism are typically absent in pseudoporphyria. Although histologically indistinguishable, the conditions differ by the finding of normal levels of porphyrins in drug-induced pseudoporphyria. Pseudoporphyria should also be differentiated from epidermolysis bullosa acquisita.

Drug-induced pseudoporphyria has been linked to numerous agents, including naproxen, nalidixic acid, tetracycline, sulfonylureas, furosemide, dapsone, pyridoxine, benoxaprofen, amiodarone, quinidine, isotretinoin, and etretinate.

Patients with juvenile rheumatoid arthritis have been noted to be particularly susceptible to naproxen-induced pseudoporphyria. In these patients, facial blisters and scarring are prominent features. Awareness of this form of phototoxicity is vital so that discontinuance of the drug might limit new blistering and subsequent irreversible facial scarring. In some cases, however, new blisters continue to develop, despite discontinuance of naproxen.

Excessive tanning parlor exposure, with or without a concomitant photosensitizer, has also been reported to precipitate pseudoporphyria.

The clinical and histologic features of PCT have also been described in hemodialysis patients. Both normal (pseudoporphyria) and elevated levels of porphyrins have been reported. Treatment with small, repeated phlebotomies, erythropoietin, deferoxamine, dialysis with high-flow rates and more permeable membranes, and transplantation has been successful.

$\mathcal{C}$linical Pearls and Pitfalls

1. Drug-induced pseudoporphyria can be distinguished from porphyria cutanea tarda by analysis of urine and stool for porphyrins and from epidermolysis bullosa acquisita by biopsy for histologic examination and immunofluorescence.

2. Naproxen-induced pseudoporphyria should be considered in the evaluation of skin complaints in patients with juvenile rheumatoid arthritis.

3. Prompt recognition of naproxen-induced pseudoporphyria and discontinuance of the medication are important to attempt to prevent further facial scarring; however, new blisters may continue to develop despite cessation of medication.

Suggested Readings

1. Carson RW, Dunnigan EJ, Dubose TD Jr, et al. Removal of plasma porphyrins with high-flux hemodialysis in porphyria cutanea tarda associated with end-stage renal disease. *J Am Soc Nephrol.* 1992;2:1445-1450,

2. Gould JW, Mercurio MG, Elmets CA, et al. Cutaneous photosensitivity diseases induced by exogenous agents. *J Am Acad Dermatol.* 1995;33:551-573.

3. Lang BA, Finlayson LA. Naproxen-induced pseudoporphyria in patients with juvenile rheumatoid arthritis. *J Pediatr.* 1994;124:639-642.

4. Stenberg A. Pseudoporphyria and sunbeds. *Acta Derm Venereol.* 1990;70:354-356.

5. Stevens BR, Fleischer AB, Piering F, et al. Porphyria cutanea tarda in the setting of renal failure: Response to renal transplantation. *Arch Dermatol.* 1993;129:337-339.

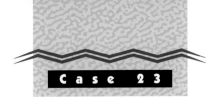
*C*hief Complaint

Nonhealing, superficial erosion in the perinasal area

*H*istory of the Present Illness

A 66-year-old Hispanic male with a 21-year history of psoriasis had received various therapies, including black tar, topical steroids, anthralin and UVB phototherapy. The disease had been controlled with outpatient UVB phototherapy two to three times per week for about 2 years, as well as topical 20% liquor carbonis detergens (LCD).

The patient presented to the Psoriasis Treatment Center with a generalized flare of plaque psoriasis of approximately 1-month duration. He reported no increased stress or infection. He did note an erosive perinasal lesion that had been present for about 3 weeks. His physician had treated the lesion for both impetigo and herpes simplex virus on an outpatient basis. The patient had received a 10-day course of dicloxacillin sodium, as well as a 10-day course of acyclovir for the lesions with minimal improvement. *Staphylococcus aureus* grew on bacterial culture; culture for herpesvirus was negative. The family history was significant for a niece who had psoriasis.

*P*hysical Examination

Physical examination revealed a well-developed, well-nourished Hispanic male with multiple, superficial, eroded lesions with irregular borders just below the nares. Widespread involvement with plaque-type psoriasis on his trunk and all extremities was also evident; the posterior lateral thighs, back, elbows, and right hand were affected. The patient's skin type was III-IV. There also was hypopigmentation accentuating the irregular plaques on the dorsum of his right hand, which he stated had been present for more than 20 years. These plaques were thought to be a combination of psoriasis and vitiligo. The patient had nail changes characteristic of psoriasis with hyperkeratosis, onychomadesis (complete shedding of the nails, usually associated with systemic disease), and oil spots on the nails. His psoriasis affected approximately 30% of the total body surface area.

The patient was admitted to the Psoriasis Day Treatment Program and Goeckerman therapy was started. Initially, the patient received 2% plain crude coal tar in petrolatum, which was gradually increased to 5% crude coal tar with 5% salicylic acid, as well as 3% anthralin and 3% salicylic acid. He also applied 0.1% triamcinolone acetonide ointment to the right hand. He tolerated up to a total of 420 millijoules of UVB light initially.

The following days were significant during the patient's therapeutic course:

- On day 4, samples were obtained from the perinasal area for bacterial cultures.

- On day 6, culture results revealed resistant *S aureus,* which was sensitive to clindamycin phosphate and trimethoprim-sulfamethoxazole. Herpes simplex virus and varicella-zoster virus cultures were negative. The patient was given a 10-day course of clindamycin (150 mg twice daily). The psoriasis continued to improve with Goeckerman treatment.

- On day 10, after finishing the course of clindamycin, the nasal lesions had not improved; a 3-mm punch biopsy was obtained just below the right nares. The decision was made to perform a biopsy because there was some concern that the patient may have a resistant herpesvirus infection with secondary immune compromise from human immunodeficiency virus (HIV) and that previous cultures for herpes were falsely negative. The patient's HIV antibody test was also negative.

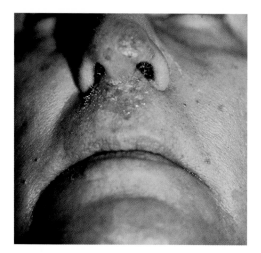

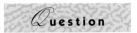

Question

*W*hat are other possible diagnoses for the nasal lesion?

Discussion

On day 15, the dermatopathology report from the perinasal lesion was interpreted as invasive squamous cell carcinoma of the perinasal area. The patient was scheduled for an appointment with the clinic for assessment for Mohs' micrographic surgery. On his initial visit, he underwent multiple repeat biopsies of the perinasal area. When the subsequent biopsies were compared with the initial biopsy, the diagnosis was changed from that of an invasive squamous cell carcinoma to mycosis fungoides, tumor stage. There was a significant amount of crush artifact from the first biopsy, which had led to a false interpretation of squamous cell carcinoma.

The patient was then referred to the mycosis fungoides clinic where he underwent a total evaluation and was thought to have some palpable right axillary lymphadenopathy. Multiple biopsies were obtained from both plaque lesions on the body and the right hand. In addition, the patient was scheduled for a total body computed tomography (CT) scan, including the chest, abdomen, and pelvis, to rule out any metastasis for mycosis fungoides.

The patient stopped attending the Psoriasis Treatment Center; phototherapy was discontinued. He underwent the total body CT scan, which revealed no evidence of metastasis. The patient also underwent a right axillary biopsy because of the axillary lymphadenopathy, which the CT scan had confirmed. The pathology diagnosis was dermatopathic lymphadenopathy, grade LN-2. Lymph nodes from mycosis fungoides patients are not considered histopathologically involved unless they are grade LN-3 or LN-4. However, mycosis fungoides cells can traffic between the skin and peripheral lymph nodes even in stage 1 disease. Multiple biopsies of plaque-like lesions on the arms, legs, chest, abdomen, and back may be necessary to confirm a diagnosis. In this case, those positive for mycosis fungoides included ones from the perinasal area and the right hand, which were previously thought to be due to psoriasis and vitiligo. The remainder of the biopsies from the trunk and extremities were positive for plaque psoriasis.

The patient is currently undergoing electron beam therapy to the perinasal and right hand lesions. Both appear to be resolving with therapy. Since the patient began electron beam therapy he has not received any phototherapy. It will be of interest to see if electron beam therapy alone will clear the patient's psoriasis as well as the mycosis lesions.

Both mycosis fungoides and psoriasis, which may appear very similar, can co-exist as papulosquamous diseases. Both are responsive to UVB phototherapy. The patient had received outpatient UVB therapy for several years. The mycosis erupted in the perinasal area where he was not receiving UVB therapy. The initial biopsy report from the perinasal area was suggestive of squamous cell carcinoma. One would think that it is important to limit exposure of this site to light. Just the opposite is the case if the lesion is mycosis fungoides. Indeed, had the patient been receiving UVB phototherapy to the face, the perinasal lesions may have been suppressed.

ℭlinical Pearls and Pitfalls

1. Mycosis fungoides and psoriasis can co-exist in some rare patients. Any suspicious lesion should be biopsied as early as possible. Numerous biopsies should be performed when there is crush artifact.

2. Both mycosis fungoides and psoriasis may respond to phototherapy, either PUVA or UVB therapy.

3. Mycosis fungoides can mimic eczema; it can also mimic psoriasis. Psoriasiform mycosis fungoides frequently has a slightly different appearance than psoriasis. Even though the plaques may be well demarcated, the scaling usually is not of micaceous quality.

Suggested Readings

1. Cooper KD. Skin-infiltrating lymphocytes in normal and disordered skin: Activation signals and functional roles in psoriasis and mycosis fungoides-type cutaneous T cell lymphoma. *J Dermatol.* 1992;11:731-737.
2. Herrmann JJ, Roenick HH Jr, Hurria A, et al. Treatment of mycosis fungoides with photochemotherapy (PUVA): Long-term follow-up. *J Am Acad Dermatol.* 1995;33(2 pt 1):234-242.
3. Honig B, Morison WL, Karp D. Photochemotherapy beyond psoriasis. *J Am Acad Dermatol.* 1994;31(5 pt 1):775-790.

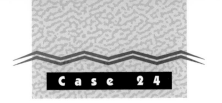

Chief Complaint

Red rash on the chest, forearms, and hands

Physical Examination

Examination showed psoriasiform and annular plaques affecting the anterior and posterior chest and extensor forearms. Coalescing pink plaques affected the dorsal hands and fingers, sparing the joints of the fingers. The face, scalp, elbows, knees, umbilicus, and sacrum were clear. The nails showed no dystrophy, but periungual telangiectasias were evident.

Biopsy for routine histology showed vacuolar alteration, edema of the papillary dermis, and an interface, as well as superficial and mid-perivascular lymphohistiocytic inflammatory cell infiltrate. Biopsy of the lesional skin for direct immunofluorescence revealed a granular, band-like pattern of IgM, IgG, and complement at the dermal-epidermal junction. Serologic findings demonstrated the presence of antinuclear, anti-Ro, and anti-La antibodies.

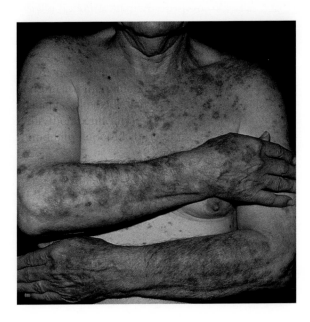

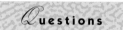

Questions

*W*hat is the differential diagnosis?

*W*hat systemic findings may be present?

*W*hat are the treatment options?

Discussion

Subacute cutaneous lupus erythematosus (SCLE) is characterized by a nonscarring, papulosquamous eruption affecting sun-exposed sites, especially the upper back and anterior chest, dorsal upper extremities, and lateral neck; the face, scalp, and lower extremities are less often involved. Patients may show a psoriasiform pattern, an annular pattern, or both. SCLE most commonly affects Caucasian women at an average age of 40 years.

The differential diagnosis of SCLE includes psoriasis, acute and discoid cutaneous lupus, dermatomyositis, phototoxic and photoallergic reactions to exogenous agents, polymorphous light eruption, granuloma annulare, and erythema multiforme. These conditions can be excluded by clinicopathologic correlation and serology. Psoriasis generally does not exacerbate with sun exposure, whereas acute lupus usually affects the face, and lesions are typically edematous with less scale than that developing with SCLE. Discoid lupus erythematosus often affects the face and scalp and often shows follicular plugging and scarring. Dermatomyositis generally affects the joints of the hands and spares interphalangeal spaces. Phototoxic reactions mimic sunburns, while photoallergic reactions and polymorphous light eruption often are manifested as edematous red papules and vesicles. Annular lesions of granuloma annulare generally demonstrate an infiltrated border. Mucosal inflammation and erosions are features of erythema multiforme.

Arthritis and arthralgias commonly affect patients with SCLE, but central nervous system disorders, renal disease, and serositis are rare features. Diseases associated with SCLE include Sjögren's, rheumatoid arthritis, and rarely, visceral malignancies, porphyria cutanea tarda, and gluten-sensitive enteropathy. Drug-induced exacerbation of SCLE has been described, particularly in association with thiazide diuretics, as well as piroxicam, procainamide, and griseofulvin. Anti-Ro antibodies are also found in association with drug-induced SCLE.

The major treatment for SCLE includes sun avoidance and protection, medium-to-potent topical corticosteroids, and antimalarial agents. Other therapies that can be considered for patients who fail to respond to conventional measures include dapsone, retinoids, azathioprine, cyclophosphamide, methotrexate, and systemic corticosteroids.

Clinical Pearls and Pitfalls

1. SCLE must be distinguished from psoriasis, photosensitive disorders, other collagen vascular diseases, granuloma annulare, and erythema multiforme.
2. Medications may be associated with the precipitation and exacerbation of SCLE. Thiazides and griseofulvin should be avoided in patients with SCLE.

Suggested Readings

1. David Bajar KM. Subacute cutaneous lupus erythematosus. *J Invest Dermatol.* 1993;100:2S-8S.
2. McCauliffe DP, Sontheimer RD. Subacute cutaneous lupus erythematosus. In: *Dublois' Lupus Erythematosus.* Philadelphia: Lea & Febiger; 1993:302-309.

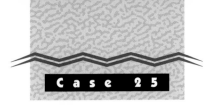
Chief Complaint

Oral warts

History of the Present Illness

A 60-year-old man presented for treatment of warts in the mouth. He reported that the lesions were slightly painful and more bothersome when he chews food. The patient has smoked two packs of cigarettes daily for the past 40 years.

Physical Examination

Examination revealed coalescing warty papules affecting the buccal mucosa along the bite line. There was no cervical adenopathy. Biopsy revealed papillomatous and endophytic bulbous epithelial hyperplasia, with evidence of some nuclear atypicality, dyskeratosis, and loss of polarity of epithelial cells.

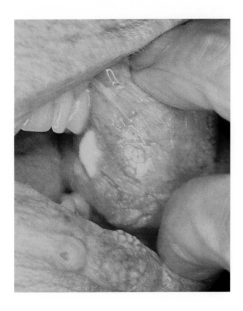

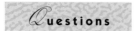

*W*hat is the diagnosis?

*W*hat is the prognosis?

*D*iscussion

Verrucous carcinoma of the oral cavity, a variant of squamous cell carcinoma, is also known as Ackerman's tumor and oral florid papillomatosis. Oral verrucous carcinoma accounts for nearly 5% to 10% of oral carcinomas, affecting primarily men in the fifth to seventh decades. Tobacco chewing and smoking are risk factors for the development of oral verrucous carcinoma. The disease usually appears as confluent white papillomas on a background of leukoplakia, most commonly along the bite line of the buccal mucosa. The gingiva is the second most common site of involvement; the hard palate, vermilion, and tongue also may be involved. Verrucous carcinoma tends to grow slowly, with significant potential for local destruction, but metastasis to regional nodes is uncommon, and distant metastasis is rare. Patients with verrucous carcinoma of the oral cavity are at increased risk for other oropharyngeal squamous cell carcinomas with more aggressive malignant behavior.

Verrucous carcinoma may affect other sites, most commonly the sole, buttock, and penis. Biopsy of papules shows superficial features resembling a verruca.

The diagnosis may be established by a large deep biopsy that reveals a bulbous endophytic epithelial extension with nuclear atypicality.

Surgical excision and Mohs' micrographic surgery are the most commonly implemented therapies for oral verrucous carcinoma. Chemotherapy also may be utilized in conjunction with excision. Radiotherapy should be avoided in most cases because of reports of subsequent anaplastic transformation and aggressive tumor behavior.

𝒞linical Pearls and Pitfalls

1. Confluent warty papules in the mouth, especially in men with a history of significant tobacco use and leukoplakia, require biopsy to rule out verrucous carcinoma.
2. The diagnosis of verrucous carcinoma necessitates a search for other oropharyngeal squamous cell carcinomas that can be expected to show more malignant behavior.
3. Radiotherapy should be considered a treatment of last resort for verrucous carcinoma because of subsequent potential for anaplastic transformation and metastases.

Suggested Reading

1. Schwartz RA. Verrucous carcinoma of the skin and mucosa. *J Am Acad Dermatol.* 1995;32:1-21.

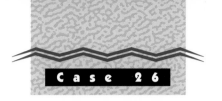

*C*hief Complaint

Tender scalp lesions

*H*istory of the Present Illness

A 40-year-old Hispanic male without significant past medical history presented with scalp lesions of 1½ years' duration and complained of recent enlargement of the lesions. The patient had visited another physician 18 months earlier, at which time a skin biopsy had been performed. This biopsy showed an acute and chronic non-specific perifollicular infiltrate. The diagnosis was most consistent with a ruptured folliculitis of the scalp. Special stains (periodic acid Schiff [PAS]) for fungi were negative. At that time, scalp treatment included triamcinolone injections and oral antibiotics (doxycycline monohydrate). The patient experienced minimal improvement with these therapies.

*P*hysical Examination and Laboratory

Physical examination revealed boggy, erythematous, scaly plaque of the left parietal scalp, 2 x 4 cm in size. The lesion was tender to palpation. A similar—though smaller (1 x 2 cm)—plaque of the right parietal scalp was evident. Areas within the plaque showed scarring alopecia. Of note, there were multiple bundles of hairs stemming from single follicular openings, giving a "hair transplant" appearance. Potassium hydroxide (KOH) testing of the lesion was negative, as was fungal culture.

Laboratory studies included a routine complete blood cell (CBC) count, liver function tests, and human immunodeficiency virus antibody testing. All study results were within normal limits. The lesions were diagnosed clinically as kerion. The patient was given oral prednisone and a 3-month course of itraconazole. After 17 days, the patient reported improvement; however, once the prednisone was tapered, he observed a worsening of both scalp lesions even though he had continued to take the full course of itraconazole.

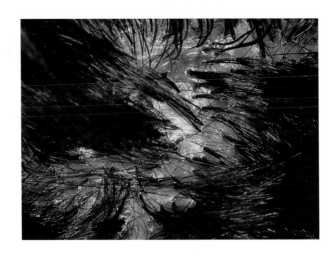

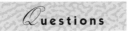

Questions

*W*hat is the diagnosis?

*W*hat treatment would be effective?

Discussion

Repeat scalp biopsy after 3 months of therapy showed a dermal, superficial perivascular and perifollicular mononuclear infiltrate. The epidermis demonstrated foci of microvesiculation and some plasma cells. Repeat PAS stain for fungi was negative. Based upon the clinical findings of multiple hairs emerging from a single follicle and a histopathologic diagnosis of folliculitis, the diagnosis of tufted folliculitis was made. The patient received a prolonged course of dicloxacillin sodium and a slow, tapering course of prednisone. He reported marked improvement in his scalp lesions within a few months of initiating the new therapy. The lesions have since stabilized.

Tufted folliculitis of the scalp was first described by Smith and Sanderson in 1978 as an area of scarring alopecia with tufts of hair emerging from a single follicular opening. Although this entity is rarely described in the literature, reported cases have shared three characteristics:

(1) An associated superficial infection caused by *Staphylococcus aureus;*

(2) Formation of tufts of hair in areas of scarring alopecia; and

(3) Focalization of fibrosis around remaining follicles.

Histologic evidence of folliculitis may be present, with several follicles converging toward a common duct. A central anagen hair may be seen, surrounded by hairs in the telogen stage of growth, which is indicated by the presence of hair bulbs and columnar cells making up the outer root sheaths. Anagen hairs are distinguished by more cuboidal cells making up the outer root sheaths.

The grouping of hair follicles or several hairs emerging from a single follicle have been described in the normal scalp. The difference between these normal "compound follicles" and pathologic tufts are the types of hairs present. A plucked hair analysis would tend to show a predominance of anagen hairs in a normal scalp, but more telogen hairs in areas of tufted folliculitis. It has been suggested that the retention of these telogen hairs over a number of hair cycles leads to tufting, which is a process associated with, but not entirely explained by, *S aureus* infection.

The patient's condition was diagnosed as kerion based upon clinical impression alone. One of the main problems in dermatologic practice is the tendency not to utilize the skin biopsy or culture as a vital diagnostic tool. When a diagnosis is made without verification, a patient may remain on ineffective treatment that can be associated with various risks. In this case, the use of an oral antifungal medication such as itraconazole requires periodic laboratory monitoring for elevated liver enzymes as an early sign of potential liver damage. In addition, the medication may interact with other medications the patient may be taking. A 3-month regimen of an oral antifungal agent is necessary before there is improvement in the condition. Without the proper diagnosis, it becomes difficult to avoid the unnecessary health risks and additional cost. Thus, although it can be difficult at times to confirm the presence of a fungal infection, treatment of suspected infection with oral antifungal agents should follow confirmation of the diagnosis by positive fungal culture and/or skin biopsy for fungal elements on PAS stain.

*C*linical Pearls and Pitfalls

1. Tufted folliculitis may resemble a scalp kerion clinically; therefore, confirmation of the diagnosis by fungal culture and/or skin biopsy is warranted.
2. Before placing a patient on a several-month regimen of therapy, it is essential to consider other unusual disease entities in the differential diagnosis.
3. If the usual therapy for a common entity has been ineffective in the past, consider less common entities as the underlying diagnosis and treat accordingly.
4. Tufted folliculitis is best treated with a combination of antibiotics to which *S aureus* is sensitive and corticosteroid therapy to reduce inflammation.

Suggested Readings

1. Smith NP, Sanderson KV. Tufted folliculitis of the scalp. *J R Soc Med*. 1978;71:606-608.

2. Luelmo-Aguilar J, Gonzalez-Castro U, Castells-Rodellas A. Tufted folliculitis: A study of four cases. *Br J Derm*. 1993;128:454-457.

3. Loewenthal LJA. "Compound" and grouped hairs of the human scalp: Their possible connection with follicular infections. *J Invest Dermatol*. 1947;8:263-273.

4. Dalziel KL, Telfer NR, Wilson CL, et al. Tufted folliculitis: A specific bacterial disease? *Am J Dermatopathol*. 1990;12(1):37-41.